Clinical Laboratory Medicine

FOR MENTAL HEALTH PROFESSIONALS

Clinical Laboratory Medicine

FOR MENTAL HEALTH PROFESSIONALS

by

Sandra A. Jacobson, M.D.

University of Arizona College of Medicine–Phoenix

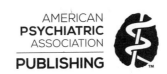

AMERICAN
PSYCHIATRIC
ASSOCIATION
PUBLISHING

If you wish to buy 50 or more copies of the same title, please go to www.appi.org/special-discounts for more information.

Copyright © 2017 American Psychiatric Association
ALL RIGHTS RESERVED

Manufactured in the United States of America on acid-free paper
22   5   4
First Edition

Typeset in Janson Text and AvantGarde.

American Psychiatric Association Publishing
1000 Wilson Boulevard
Arlington, VA 22209-3901
www.appi.org

Library of Congress Cataloging-in-Publication Data
Names: Jacobson, Sandra A., author. | Abridgement of (work): Jacobson, Sandra A., Laboratory medicine in psychiatry and behavioral science. | American Psychiatric Association, issuing body.
Title: Clinical laboratory medicine for mental health professionals / by Sandra A. Jacobson.
Description: First edition. | Arlington, Virginia : American Psychiatric Association Publishing, [2017] | Abridgement of Laboratory medicine in psychiatry and behavioral science / by Sandra A. Jacobson. 1st ed. Washington, D.C. : American Psychiatric Pub., c2012. | Includes bibliographical references and index.
Identifiers: LCCN 2016046721 (print) | LCCN 2016047207 (ebook) | ISBN 9781615370849 (pbk. : alk. paper) | ISBN 9781615371211 (ebook)
Subjects: | MESH: Mental Disorders—diagnosis | Clinical Laboratory Techniques | Psychotropic Drugs—analysis
Classification: LCC RC456 (print) | LCC RC456 (ebook) | NLM WM 141 | DDC 616.89—dc23
LC record available at https://lccn.loc.gov/2016046721

British Library Cataloguing in Publication Data
A CIP record is available from the British Library.

Contents

CHAPTER 1

CHAPTER 2

Diseases and Conditions. 179

CHAPTER 3

Psychotropic Medications: Laboratory Screening and Monitoring. 239

Appendix. 277

References 287

Index 295

Preface

Clinical Laboratory Medicine for Mental Health Professionals had its origin in the pages of the earlier reference work, *Clinical Manual of Laboratory Medicine in Psychiatry and Behavioral Science* (published in 2012). The current work is abridged to focus more directly on the needs of general psychiatric practice, and it also has been revised and updated from the earlier work.

Like its predecessor, *Clinical Laboratory Medicine for Mental Health Professionals* is designed to assist psychiatrists and other behavioral health clinicians in the care of psychiatric inpatients, outpatients, day hospital patients, general medical/surgical patients seen in consultation in the general hospital, and geriatric or disabled patients in long-term care settings. The book does not have a focus on child psychiatry and does not cover the care of neonates or infants.

To facilitate its use as a reference manual, the book is divided into three chapters:

- Laboratory Tests
- Diseases and Conditions
- Psychotropic Medications: Laboratory Screening and Monitoring

Each of the three chapters is organized alphabetically. The book is also extensively indexed.

Among the thousands of laboratory tests available, those selected for inclusion met one or more of the following criteria: a core or basic laboratory test for any patient; one that was particularly pertinent to psychiatry or behavioral health; or one that was new to medicine and potentially of interest in the field of behavioral health, including geriatrics. Diseases and conditions selected for inclusion were those for which laboratory tests are primary or important in diagnosis or differential diagnosis; those that are core or common conditions among psychiatric patients or geriatric psychiatry patients; or those that have important psychiatric, cognitive, or behavioral consequences.

Years of clinical practice and research in neuropsychiatry inform not only the choice of tests but also the rationale for their use. A large number of published sources were consulted, including reference texts (e.g., *Harrison's Principles of Internal Medicine*, 19th Edition [Kasper et al. 2015] and others), reference manuals (e.g., *Tietz Clinical Guide to Laboratory Tests*, 4th Edition [Wu 2006] and others), handbooks (e.g., *Handbook of Medical Psychiatry*, 2nd Edition [Moore and Jefferson 2004]), Internet sources (e.g., ARUP Laboratories' Test Directory [ARUP Laboratories 2010] at www.aruplab.com and Mayo Medical Laboratories Test Catalog [Mayo Clinic 2016] at www.mayomedicallaboratories.com), and primary and review references from the medical literature accessed through PubMed. A complete listing may be found in the "References" section at the end of the book.

References

ARUP Laboratories: Laboratory Test Directory. Available at: http://www.aruplab.com. Accessed May 2010.

Kasper DL, Fauci AS, Hauser SL, et al (eds): Harrison's Principles of Internal Medicine, 19th Edition. New York, McGraw-Hill, 2015

Mayo Clinic: Mayo Medical Laboratories Test Catalog. Available at: http://www.mayomedical-laboratories.com/test-catalog/. Accessed May–August 2016.

Moore DP, Jefferson JW: Handbook of Medical Psychiatry, 2nd Edition. Philadelphia, PA, Elsevier/Mosby, 2004

Wu AHB: Tietz Clinical Guide to Laboratory Tests, 4th Edition. St. Louis, MO, WB Saunders, 2006

Introduction

General Guidelines for Laboratory Testing

Judicious use of the laboratory improves patient care in psychiatry and behavioral science, just as it does in all other branches of medicine. Laboratory testing is only one component of the complete evaluation, which also includes a history, review of systems, functional assessment, and physical and mental status examinations. When laboratory results are reviewed in the context of the patient's family history, personal history, lifestyle, and particular exam findings, there is less likelihood of overreacting to a result that may turn out to be spurious. For example, with an isolated elevation in one test such as alanine transaminase (ALT) and in the absence of any clinical evidence of disease, the test should simply be repeated and further workup performed only if a twofold or greater elevation persists. When laboratory findings are unclear or introduce questions, clinical laboratory staff can be an excellent resource for clinicians in the interpretation of test data and in planning an approach to a diagnostic evaluation that includes the laboratory.

The reference ranges cited in the text are only general guides. Few reference ranges apply across laboratories and testing methods. Reference intervals supplied by the testing laboratory supersede the intervals suggested in this work. It is critical that the clinician pay close attention to the units of measurement to avoid, for example, confusing measures such as μg (microgram) and mg (milligram).

Laboratory Testing in Psychiatry

What constitutes standard laboratory screening for psychiatric patients in general is not well established. Indeed, the American Psychiatric Association *Practice Guidelines for the Treatment of Psychiatric Disorders* (2000) suggest only that laboratory testing is used to establish or exclude a diagnosis, direct choice of treatment, or to monitor treatment effects or side effects. Unfortunately, the updated practice guidelines (American Psychiatric Association 2016) reflect an outright skepticism as to the value of laboratory testing in psychiatry, recommending that "the decision to do laboratory studies and other clinical tests, such as imaging studies, electrocardiography (ECG), or electroencephalography (EEG), should be based on the likelihood that the test result will alter diagnostic or treatment-related decision making." Surely this is not the standard of medical practice in psychiatry in this millennium.

Not surprisingly, clinical practice varies in terms of what laboratory tests are ordered and how often these "labs" are checked. There does appear to be general agreement that a screening laboratory evaluation is indicated for the following categories of patients: those presenting for the first time with major psychiatric syndromes (e.g., psychosis or major mood disorder), elderly patients admitted to the hospital, patients who are undernourished or dehydrated, patients with alcohol or drug dependence, and those with delirium or initial presentation of dementia.

Patients admitted to inpatient psychiatry services may undergo the following laboratory evaluation upon admission:

- Complete blood count (CBC)
- Comprehensive metabolic panel (CMP)
- Urinalysis
- Urine drug screen with alcohol
- HIV testing (from which patients may "opt out")

For patients at risk of metabolic syndrome, or those who are being started on an atypical antipsychotic drug, the following may be added:

- Lipid panel
- Hemoglobin A_{1C}

Thyroid-stimulating hormone (TSH) may be checked for patients presenting with mood disorders or significant anxiety, and for all women over 50 years, unless TSH was tested within the last year. Sexually transmitted infection screening may be performed for those with a history of substance abuse, Cluster B personality disorder (antisocial, borderline, histrionic, narcissistic), or bipolar disorder. Urine or serum pregnancy testing may be performed if there is any question of pregnancy. More extensive laboratory testing may be indicated for patients presenting with syndromes such as acute psychosis, as discussed in Chapter 2, "Diseases and Conditions."

■ Electrocardiogram

Inpatient psychiatrists and those working in research settings may be required to obtain and provide preliminary interpretation of electrocardiogram (ECG) tracings. The ECG is covered in Chapter 1, "Laboratory Tests," and the Appendix includes a table listing 10 rules for a normal ECG and a figure reviewing waves and intervals on the ECG.

■ Chemistries

The largest component of the chapter on laboratory tests is *blood chemistries*. These are the laboratory tests most often found to be abnormal in patients seen in consultation in the general hospital, and also often contribute to the assessment for delirium in this setting.

■ Genetic Testing

Genetic tests that are covered in this work include apolipoprotein E (ApoE) genotyping and cytochrome P450 (CYP450) genotyping. Useful information about other genetic tests and associated diseases can be found at the National Institutes of Health–associated Web site www.genetests.org. For most clinicians, genetic tests will be laboratory "send-outs," and it will be important to inquire directly with the receiving laboratory about costs before sending samples, as this testing can be prohibitively expensive and not covered by existing insurance policies.

■ Hematology

Basic hematology is relevant to psychiatric practice not only because hematologic abnormalities may underlie symptoms such as fatigue and inattention, but also because psychotropic medications may significantly affect hematologic values. Tests covered include complete blood count (CBC), hemoglobin, hematocrit, mean corpuscular volume (MCV), platelet count, red blood cell count (RBC), and white blood cell count (WBC).

■ Imaging

Neuroimaging is a core component of the diagnostic workup for a variety of conditions at the interface of psychiatry and neurology. Imaging is indicated when signs and symptoms of a major psychiatric disorder first become manifest, for atypical presentations, for unusual age at onset, or for psychiatric symptoms associated with a focal neurological examination. Basic neuroimaging modalities covered in this work include cranial computed tomography (CT), brain magnetic resonance imaging (MRI), positron emission tomography (PET), and single photon emission computed tomography (SPECT).

■ Psychotropic Medications

Chapter 3 covers laboratory screening and monitoring—"safety labs"—pertinent to psychotropic medications. Chapter 1 includes information about drug level testing for a selected group of medications, including benzodiazepines, carbamazepine, clozapine, lithium, and valproate.

The Appendix includes a table summarizing therapeutic and toxic drug levels for commonly used psychotropic medications.

Reference

American Psychiatric Association, Work Group on Psychiatric Evaluation: The American Psychiatric Association Practice Guidelines for the Psychiatric Evaluation of Adults, 3rd Edition. Arlington, VA, American Psychiatric Association, 2016. Available at: http://psychiatryonline.org/doi/pdf/10.1176/appi.books.9780890426760. Accessed September 4, 2016.

About the Author

Sandra Jacobson received her medical degree from the John A. Burns School of Medicine in her home state of Hawaii. After completing an internship in internal medicine at the University of Hawaii Integrated Medical Residency Program in Honolulu, she underwent psychiatry residency training and fellowship training in neurophysiology at UCLA Neuropsychiatric Institute. She has held faculty positions at UCLA, Tufts University School of Medicine, the Warren Alpert School of Medicine at Brown University, and the University of Arizona College of Medicine–Phoenix. Her work in consultation/liaison psychiatry, inpatient and outpatient psychiatry, geriatric psychiatry, nursing home consultation, and clinical neurophysiology (electroencephalography) informs the format, choice of tests and diseases, and comments on psychiatric relevance for the material included in this manual.

CHAPTER 1

Laboratory Tests

Alanine transaminase (ALT)	
Type of test	Blood
Explanation of test	ALT is an enzyme localized mostly to the liver. Under normal conditions, ALT levels in blood are low. When the liver is injured, ALT is released into the circulation and provides an early sign of this injury before clinical symptoms develop. Extreme elevations of ALT (>10× normal) usually suggest acute hepatitis, often viral in origin. In this condition, ALT levels can remain high for as long as 6 months. In chronic hepatitis, on the other hand, ALT levels may be only minimally elevated (<4× normal) or even high-normal. The most common cause of mild ALT elevation in the Western Hemisphere is nonalcoholic fatty liver disease. In liver disease such as cirrhosis or biliary obstruction, ALT levels may be normal. ALT values are usually considered in relation to other liver function tests (LFTs), such as aspartate transaminase (AST) and alkaline phosphatase (ALP). In alcoholic liver disease, the ratio of AST to ALT is high (2:1 or more), even when neither value is elevated. AST is more sensitive to alcoholic liver disease, but ALT is more specific. In extrahepatic biliary obstruction, ALT is usually more elevated than AST. In acute myocardial infarction, AST is always elevated, but ALT is not unless there is also liver injury.
Relevance to psychiatry and behavioral science	ALT is one of the tests of liver health (liver "function") that is closely monitored in psychiatric practice, mainly because of the potential hepatotoxicity of psychotropic drugs. ALT is also monitored in patients with alcoholism, substance-induced liver disease, and hepatitis. Elevation of ALT may be found on routine screening. If the patient has no clinical symptoms and no risk factors for liver disease, and ALT is less than three times the upper limit of normal (ULN), a recheck is indicated after 1–3 months. If the elevation persists, further investigation is needed. If ALT is >3× ULN on a single measurement, further investigation is needed. Elevation of ALT may occur with initiation of a new psychotropic medication. In most cases, the ALT increase is benign, and the lab value will revert to baseline within weeks of dose stabilization. Further investigation is needed in cases where the value does not normalize or when ALP or bilirubin is also elevated.

Alanine transaminase (ALT) *(continued)*

Relevance to psychiatry and behavioral science *(continued)*	Pathological elevation of ALT may occur with alcoholism, substance-induced liver disease, and hepatitis. It is important not to be misled by a normal ALT value in a patient with established cirrhosis. In the patient with cirrhosis due to hepatitis C with a normal ALT result, active hepatitis may be present, such that the patient would benefit from antiviral therapy, beta-blockers to prevent variceal bleeding, and other treatments. AST and ALT levels may also be normal in patients with hemochromatosis, in patients taking methotrexate, or after jejunoileal bypass surgery, despite advanced liver disease. In all cases, the patient's history should be taken into account, and an effort should be made to identify other evidence of liver disease.
Preparation of patient	None needed
Indications	• A component of the LFT panel • A component of the comprehensive metabolic panel • Monitoring medication effects on the liver (see Appendix). • Clinical symptoms of liver disease, such as jaundice, abdominal pain, ascites, nausea, vomiting, or darkening of the urine • Distinguishing hemolytic jaundice from jaundice due to liver dysfunction • Evaluating patients with hepatitis exposure or symptoms of hepatitis • Evaluating patients with alcoholism or other substance abuse • Monitoring the effects of treatment for liver disease
Reference range	Males: 10–40 U/L (0.17–0.68 mkat/L) Females: 7–35 U/L (0.12–0.60 mkat/L) Normal values may vary with testing method.
Critical value(s)	>300 IU/L indicates acute hepatic injury
Increased levels	• Acute viral, infectious, ischemic, or toxic hepatitis (30–50× normal) • Hepatic necrosis due to drugs (e.g., acetaminophen) • Hepatocellular disease (moderate to marked increase) • Alcoholic cirrhosis (mild increase) • Metastatic liver disease (mild increase)

Alanine transaminase (ALT) *(continued)*	
Increased levels *(continued)*	• Biliary obstruction (mild increase) • Fatty liver (mild increase) • Mild increase (<1.5× ULN) can be normal for gender, ethnicity, or body mass index.
Decreased levels	Certain drugs can falsely decrease levels.
Interfering factors	Levels are normally slightly higher in males and African Americans. Many psychotropic drugs can falsely elevate ALT values. Aspirin, interferon, phenothiazines, and simvastatin can falsely reduce ALT values.
Cross-references	Alcohol Use Disorder (Alcoholism) Aspartate Transaminase (AST) Fatty Liver Disease (Nonalcoholic) Hepatitis (Viral) Hy's Law (see Figure 2 in Appendix) Liver Function Tests (LFTs)

Gopal DV, Rosen HR: Abnormal findings on liver function tests: interpreting results to narrow the diagnosis and establish a prognosis. Postgrad Med 107:100–102, 105–109, 113–114, 2000

Theal RM, Scott K: Evaluating asymptomatic patients with abnormal liver function test results. Am Fam Physician 53(6):2111–2119, 1996

Albumin	
Type of test	Blood
Explanation of test	The most abundant protein in plasma, albumin serves primarily to maintain oncotic pressure inside blood vessels to keep them from becoming "leaky." It has a similar function in the urinary tract and cerebrospinal fluid. In addition, albumin transports various drugs and nutrients, provides a source of nourishment for tissues, and contributes to an acid-base buffer system in the blood. Albumin is normally reabsorbed in the kidneys, such that undetectable levels are found in urine. The presence of albumin in the urine (as microalbumin or protein) presages or indicates abnormal kidney function. Albumin may also be lost from the blood through the gastrointestinal tract or skin or because of hemorrhage.
Relevance to psychiatry and behavioral science	Albumin has numerous basic physiological functions, and it is routinely checked as part of the comprehensive metabolic panel. The albumin level may be low in states of malnutrition, such as anorexia nervosa or failure to thrive, and in alcoholism with cirrhosis. The albumin level is also of importance in psychopharmacology in managing the use of highly protein-bound drugs. When the albumin level is low, the unbound percentage of these drugs is high, and the measured concentration of total drug may underestimate the amount of drug acting on the target organ. In this case, the patient could develop symptoms of toxicity at apparently therapeutic levels. Free drug levels, which are available for many psychotropics, can be helpful in this situation.
Preparation of patient	None needed
Indications	• Evaluating nutritional status (prealbumin preferred) • Evaluating liver disease • Evaluating kidney disease • Determining the effects of hemorrhage, burns, or defects in the gastrointestinal tract
Reference range	Adults: 3.5–5.2 g/dL (35–52 g/L) Children: 3.8–5.4 g/dL (38–54 g/L)
Critical value(s)	<1.5 g/dL (<15 g/L) Levels of 2.0–2.5 g/dL may be associated with edema.
Increased levels	• Dehydration • *Drugs:* anabolic steroids, androgens, growth hormones, and insulin

Albumin *(continued)*	
Decreased levels	• Liver damage, cirrhosis, alcoholism
	• Nephrotic syndrome, renal disease
	• Inflammatory bowel disease (Crohn's disease, colitis)
	• Heart failure
	• Burns
	• Severe skin disease
	• Undernutrition, starvation, malabsorption, anorexia
	• Acute inflammation (a "negative" acute-phase reactant)
	• Chronic inflammation
	• Thyroid disease: Cushing disease, thyrotoxicosis
	• Prolonged hospitalization or bed rest
	• *Drugs:* estrogens
Interfering factors	Level declines slowly after age 40 years. Decreased albumin levels occur in the last trimester of pregnancy. Intravenous fluids may invalidate results because of dilutional effects.
Cross-references	Alcohol Use Disorder (Alcoholism)
	Anorexia Nervosa
	Comprehensive Metabolic Panel (CMP)
	Eating Disorders
	Protein

Boldt J: Use of albumin: an update. Br J Anaesth 104(3):276–284, 2010

Alkaline phosphatase (ALP)	
Type of test	Blood
Explanation of test	ALP is an enzyme concentrated in osteoblasts (bone-forming cells) and cells that form the bile canaliculi in the liver. Smaller amounts of ALP are found in the placenta and bowel. Each of these organs elaborates a different isoenzyme of ALP that can be distinguished by fractionation. Total ALP levels are used to evaluate liver and bone disease, with high levels indicating tissue injury.
	When ALP is elevated in tandem with other liver function tests, such as aspartate transaminase (AST), alanine transaminase (ALT), or bilirubin, the cause of the ALP elevation is usually hepatic. In liver disease such as biliary obstruction, ALP and bilirubin are increased out of proportion to increases in AST or ALT. In hepatocellular liver injury such as occurs in hepatitis, ALT and AST are increased out of proportion to ALP. If the ALP level is high and the source of the elevation is unknown, ALP can be fractionated, or gamma-glutamyltransferase (GGT) can be assayed. GGT is another enzyme produced in the liver that is not made by bone. GGT elevation then indicates a hepatic source.
	If ALP is elevated and calcium and phosphate levels are abnormal, the cause is usually bone related. Cancer metastatic to bone or liver can cause elevation in ALP. With treatment, ALP levels may decline. In some bone diseases such as Paget disease, ALP may be the only laboratory abnormality, and the elevation seen can be up to 25 times the normal value. ALP is elevated in osteomalacia but not osteoporosis, so the value can help distinguish these conditions.
Relevance to psychiatry and behavioral science	Numerous psychotropic drugs are associated with increased ALP levels (see "Interfering Factors," below).
	ALP elevation may be found on routine screening.
	• If ALP is <1.5 times the upper limit of normal (ULN), recheck in 1–3 months.
	• If ALP is >1.5× ULN on two measurements 6 months apart, further investigation is needed.
	• If ALP is >3× ULN on a single measurement, further investigation is needed.
	A cholestatic drug reaction is suggested by an increase in ALP, usually >3 times the ULN. AST and ALT levels are normal or only minimally elevated (see Figure 3 in Appendix). Alcoholism and cirrhosis are both associated with ALP elevation. In alcohol-related hepatitis, the ALP elevation is <2× ULN, and it does not correlate well with bilirubin level.

Alkaline phosphatase (ALP) *(continued)*	
Preparation of patient	Overnight fasting before the test is preferred because enzyme activity is affected by eating, especially fatty food.
Indications	• A component of the liver function test panel • Signs/symptoms of liver disease • Signs/symptoms of bone disease
Reference range	Adults: 25–100 U/L (0.43–1.70 µkat/L) Children 1–12 years: <350 U/L (<5.95 µkat/L) Males 12–14 years: <500 U/L (<8.50 µkat/L) The reference range for ALP in children is different from that for adults because ALP is elevated during active bone growth.
Critical value(s)	None
Increased levels	• Liver diseases: cirrhosis, alcoholism, hepatitis, cholestasis, cancer (primary or metastatic), infectious mononucleosis, diabetes, Gilbert syndrome • Bone diseases: cancer (primary or metastatic), Paget disease, osteomalacia, rickets, osteogenesis imperfecta • Hyperparathyroidism (with elevated calcium) • Hyperthyroidism • Infarction (myocardial or pulmonary) • Hodgkin disease • Lung or pancreatic cancer • Ulcerative colitis • Peptic ulcer disease • Amyloidosis • Sarcoidosis • Bowel infarction or perforation • Chronic renal failure • Congestive heart failure
Decreased levels	• Hypothyroidism • Pernicious anemia and other anemias • Malnutrition • Magnesium or zinc deficiency • Milk-alkali syndrome • Celiac sprue • Congenital hypophosphatasia

Alkaline phosphatase (ALP) *(continued)*	
Interfering factors	ALP levels increase at room temperature and in refrigeration; tests should be run the same day as collection. ALP levels decrease if blood is anticoagulated. People over 50 years of age may have 1.5 times the normal level of ALP without pathology. Growing bones in children cause high ALP levels, with large increases seen during growth spurts in puberty. Elevated ALP levels are seen in pregnancy and after menopause. ALP levels increase after fatty meals. Elevation in ALP is seen for several days after albumin infusion. A very large number of drugs are associated with ALP elevation, including all psychotropic drug classes and nearly all members of each class.
Cross-references	Alcohol Use Disorder (Alcoholism) Cholestatic Drug Reaction (see Figure 3 in Appendix) Cirrhosis Liver Function Tests (LFTs)

Corathers SD: Focus on diagnosis: the alkaline phosphatase level: nuances of a familiar test. Pediatr Rev 27(10):382–384, 2006

Giannini EG, Testa R, Savarino V: Liver enzyme alteration: a guide for clinicians. CMAJ 172(3):367–379, 2005

Padda MS, Sanchez M, Akhtar AJ, Boyer JL: Drug induced cholestasis. Hepatology 53:1377–1387, 2011

Reust CE, Hall L: Clinical inquiries. What is the differential diagnosis of an elevated alkaline phosphatase (AP) level in an otherwise asymptomatic patient? J Fam Pract 50(6):496–497, 2001

Alprazolam level	
Type of test	Blood
Explanation of test	Benzodiazepines are Schedule IV sedative-hypnotic drugs used to treat anxiety and insomnia. Alprazolam is a fast- to intermediate-acting drug with a half-life that varies considerably among individual patients. In general, levels are checked when either overdose or noncompliance is suspected or to detect use without a prescription. Although illicit use of a benzodiazepine is usually checked with a urine drug screen, many urine assays for benzodiazepines target drugs that are metabolized to either oxazepam or nordiazepam and are thus insensitive to alprazolam.
Relevance to psychiatry and behavioral science	Toxicity with chronic benzodiazepine ingestion may be manifested as confusion, disorientation, memory impairment, ataxia, decreased reflexes, and dysarthria. With acute overdose, the patient may exhibit somnolence, confusion, ataxia, decreased reflexes, vertigo, dysarthria, respiratory depression, and coma. More serious consequences usually involve co-ingestion of alcohol or other sedatives. If the ingestion was within 4 hours or if the patient is symptomatic, activated charcoal should be given and then repeated, as these drugs undergo hepatic recirculation. Administration of flumazenil does not affect drug level.
Preparation of patient	None needed
Indications	• Screening for drug use • Suspicion of overdose • Signs of toxicity in a treated patient • Suspected noncompliance with prescribed therapy
Reference range	10–40 ng/mL with low-dose therapy (1–4 mg daily) 50–100 ng/mL with high-dose therapy (6–9 mg daily)
Critical value(s)	Above upper limits noted
Increased levels	• Overdose • Overuse • Poor metabolism • Hepatic encephalopathy
Decreased levels	Noncompliance
Interfering factors	None
Cross-reference	Benzodiazepines

Galanter M, Kleber HD, Brady KT (eds): The American Psychiatric Publishing Textbook of Substance Abuse Treatment, 5th Edition. Arlington, VA, American Psychiatric Publishing, 2015

Ammonia (NH₃)

Type of test	Blood
Explanation of test	Ammonia is a waste product made by intestinal bacteria and other cells in the course of protein digestion. Under normal conditions, it is transformed in the liver to urea, which can be excreted by the kidneys. If this cycle malfunctions, ammonia can build up in the blood, affecting acid-base balance and brain function. In acute hepatic failure, with a rapid rise in ammonia levels, there is a reasonable correlation of venous with arterial ammonia levels and of arterial ammonia with brain glutamine levels.
Relevance to psychiatry and behavioral science	Routine blood tests do not include ammonia assays. Unless there is clinical suspicion of ammonia elevation based on the patient's history or exam findings, the ammonia level is not checked. For this reason, hyperammonemia is likely to be underdiagnosed in many settings. Elevated ammonia levels can be found in hepatic failure due to alcoholic cirrhosis, hepatitis, and Wilson disease, among other conditions. Acute hyperammonemia is associated with delirium and other mental status changes as well as seizures. In severe cases, coma and death from brain herniation can supervene. When acute hyperammonemia is suspected, the ammonia level should be checked and ordered *stat*, because this represents a medically urgent situation. The *stat* order is also critical to the accuracy of the test, because ammonia levels increase with the breakdown of proteins during blood storage. Chronic hyperammonemia has less severe effects because of compensatory effects in ammonia metabolism and dampening of excitatory effects on the brain.
Preparation of patient	If possible, the patient should fast except for water for 8 hours before the test. The patient should not smoke for 2 hours before the test.
Indications	• Workup for mental status changes • Workup for lethargy and vomiting in a child after viral illness • Diagnosing hepatic encephalopathy • Diagnosing Reye syndrome • Monitoring severity of hepatic disease and response to treatment • Evaluating genetic urea cycle disorders • Monitoring patients on hyperalimentation

Ammonia (NH₃) *(continued)*

Reference range	Check lab report to determine assay (NH₃ or N).
	
	Measured as NH₃
	    Adults: 15–60 µg/dL (11–35 µmol/L)
	    Higher levels from birth up to 2 years
	
	Measured as N
	    Adults: 15–45 µg/dL (11–32 µmol/L)
	    Higher levels in infants

Critical value(s)	NH₃ >200 µmol/L
Increased levels	• Liver disease, especially after a precipitant such as gastrointestinal bleeding or electrolyte imbalance • Decreased blood flow to the liver • Gastrointestinal hemorrhage • Gastrointestinal tract infection with distention and stasis • Reye syndrome (with decreased glucose levels) • Renal failure • Total parenteral nutrition • Heritable defects in urea cycle enzymes (can appear at any age) • *Drugs:* alcohol, valproate, barbiturates, diuretics, and opioids
Decreased levels	• Hypertension • Antibiotics such as neomycin
Interfering factors	Sampling techniques greatly affect ammonia values. Hemolysis, use of a tight tourniquet, clenching the fist, or allowing the sample to sit increases ammonia levels. Exercise or other muscular exertion increases ammonia levels. Smoking increases ammonia levels.
Cross-references	Alcohol Use Disorder (Alcoholism) Hepatic Encephalopathy Hepatitis (Viral)

Cohn RM, Roth KS: Hyperammonemia, bane of the brain. Clin Pediatr (Phila) 43(8):683–689, 2004

Kundra A, Jain A, Banga A, et al: Evaluation of plasma ammonia levels in patients with acute liver failure and chronic liver disease and its correlation with the severity of hepatic encephalopathy and clinical features of raised intracranial tension. Clin Biochem 38(8):696–699, 2005

Amylase

Type of test	Blood
Explanation of test	Amylase is an enzyme produced by the parotid glands and the pancreas that facilitates digestion of complex carbohydrates. Amylase is excreted by the kidneys. It enters the circulation in large amounts when the salivary glands or pancreas are inflamed. The most important use of amylase testing is to diagnose acute pancreatitis, although lipase is more specific for this condition. In acute pancreatitis, the serum amylase level begins to rise 2 hours after onset, peaks at 24 hours, and persists for 2–4 days. Amylase appears in the urine with a lag time of 6–10 hours and persists for 7–10 days.

Amylase can also be high in macroamylasemia. In this condition, amylase is bound to immunoglobulin, forming a molecule that is poorly filtered by the kidney because of its large size. Macroamylasemia does not cause symptoms, but it is associated with other diseases, such as ulcerative colitis, celiac disease, HIV infection, and rheumatoid arthritis. It is also seen in apparently healthy patients. Macroamylasemia can be distinguished from acute pancreatitis by measuring urine amylase, which is low in macroamylasemia and high in acute pancreatitis. |
Relevance to psychiatry and behavioral science	Amylase is elevated along with lipase in pancreatitis, and certain populations are at particular risk for this condition, including patients with alcoholism (especially males), gallstones (especially females), and hyperlipidemia and those treated with medications such as valproate, corticosteroids, or isoniazid (INH). Amylase of salivary origin may be elevated in patients with eating disorders that include purging behaviors.
Preparation of patient	The patient should fast for at least 2 hours before the test.
Indications	Used with lipase for the following indications: • Diagnosing acute pancreatitis • Monitoring treatment for acute pancreatitis • Distinguishing pancreatitis from other abdominal disorders
Reference range	Adults ≤60 years: 25–125 U/L (0.4–2.1 μkat/L) Adults >60 years: 24–151 U/L (0.4–2.5 μkat/L)
Critical value(s)	None

Amylase *(continued)*	
Increased levels	• Pancreatitis
	• Other pancreatic disease or trauma
	• Eating disorder with purging
	• Partial gastrectomy
	• Appendicitis, peritonitis
	• Perforated peptic ulcer
	• Traumatic brain injury
	• Shock
	• Mumps or other salivary gland/duct inflammation or obstruction
	• Acute cholecystitis (stone in the common bile duct)
	• Intestinal obstruction
	• Ruptured ectopic pregnancy
	• Macroamylasemia
	• *Drugs:* clozapine, desipramine, donepezil, mirtazapine, risperidone, valproate, and numerous other nonpsychotropic medications, including acetaminophen, nonsteroidal anti-inflammatory drugs, many opioids, and steroids
Decreased levels	• Pancreatic insufficiency, pancreatectomy
	• Liver disease, hepatitis
	• Cystic fibrosis
	• *Drugs:* anabolic steroids, cefotaxime, propylthiouracil, zidovudine, and others
Interfering factors	Anticoagulated blood and lipemic serum are interfering factors. Pregnancy and diabetes increase levels.
Cross-reference	Lipase

Ghio L, Fornaro G, Rossi P: Risperidone-induced hyperamylasemia, hyperlipasemia, and neuroleptic malignant syndrome: a case report. J Clin Psychopharmacol 29(4):391–392, 2009

Antinuclear antibody (ANA) test	
Type of test	Blood
Explanation of test	The ANA test screens for systemic rheumatic diseases, including systemic lupus erythematosus (SLE), rheumatoid arthritis, polymyositis/dermatomyositis, mixed connective tissue disease, Sjögren syndrome, scleroderma, and CREST syndrome. The ANA result is reported as a titer, along with the immunofluorescence pattern when the titer is high enough to be considered positive. In general, a titer of 1:160 or more is considered positive (>3 on enzyme-linked immunosorbent assay [ELISA]), although some experts use the more stringent threshold of 1:320 to indicate positivity.
	When a high titer is obtained with screening, an extractable nuclear antigen (ENA) antibody panel can help to identify the specific disease:
	• Presence of anti–double-stranded DNA and anti-Smith (anti-Sm) antibodies in SLE
	• Anti-histone antibodies in drug-induced lupus
	• Anti–single-stranded-A antibodies (Ro) and anti–single-stranded-B antibodies (La) in Sjögren syndrome
	• Positive anticentromere test, presence of anti–Scl-70 antibodies in scleroderma
	The immunofluorescence pattern also may be helpful in identifying the specific disease:
	• Homogeneous (diffuse) pattern: SLE and mixed connective tissue disease
	• Speckled pattern: SLE, Sjögren syndrome, scleroderma, polymyositis, rheumatoid arthritis, and mixed connective tissue disease
	• Nucleolar pattern: scleroderma and polymyositis
	• Outline (peripheral) pattern: SLE
	The diagnosis of a systemic rheumatic disease is based on clinical signs and symptoms, and these tests are used only to confirm the diagnosis and identify the specific disease.

Antinuclear antibody (ANA) test *(continued)*

Relevance to psychiatry and behavioral science	The ANA test is most often used to diagnose SLE (lupus). This is the most common autoimmune connective tissue disease in pediatrics. The condition can also appear in adults, even in late life, although most patients become symptomatic between puberty and age 40. Common neuropsychiatric symptoms of lupus include headaches, anxiety disorders, mood disorders, psychosis, cognitive dysfunction, and delirium. Seizures, abnormal movements (chorea, dystonia, hemiballismus), and stroke can occur. Drug-induced lupus can also cause a positive test and is important to rule out, because this condition will subside when the offending drug is discontinued. Psychotropic medications associated with drug-induced lupus include carbamazepine, oxcarbazepine, phenytoin, and sertraline. Nonpsychotropics include hydralazine, isoniazid (INH), and procainamide.
Preparation of patient	None needed
Indications	• Symptoms suggestive of autoimmune disease: low-grade fever, joint pain, fatigue, and/or rash • Suspicion of a second autoimmune disease in an affected patient • Unexplained neuropsychiatric symptoms
Reference range	≥1:160 on immunofluorescence antibody testing >3 on ELISA testing
Critical value(s)	None
Positive test	SLE Drug-induced lupus Sjögren syndrome Scleroderma Rheumatoid arthritis Raynaud disease Dermatomyositis Mixed connective tissue disease
Negative test	The patient is unlikely to have one of these autoimmune disorders, although the test may need to be repeated at a later time because of the intermittent nature of these diseases.

Antinuclear antibody (ANA) test *(continued)*

Interfering factors	False positives are more likely when titer ≤1:160.
	False positives are seen in 3%–5% of Caucasians, in 10%–37% of patients over age 65 years, and with certain drugs and infections.
	A false-positive result can be seen in primary antiphospholipid syndrome.
Cross-references	None

Hanly JG, Urowitz MB, Siannis F, et al; Systemic Lupus International Collaborating Clinics: Autoantibodies and neuropsychiatric events at the time of systemic lupus erythematosus diagnosis: results from an international inception cohort study. Arthritis Rheum 58(3):843–853, 2008

Katz U, Zandman-Goddard G: Drug-induced lupus: an update. Autoimmun Rev 10(1):46–50, 2010

Apolipoprotein E (ApoE) genotyping

Type of test	Blood
Explanation of test	Although the role of the ApoE ε4 allele in the pathogenesis of Alzheimer's disease (AD) is not completely known, an association of the ε4 allele with amyloid plaque burden has been described. Of the three ApoE alleles—ε2, ε3, and ε4—the most common is ε3, which is present in more than 50% of the general population. The ε4 allele is a risk factor for the development of sporadic or familial late-onset AD, while the ε2 allele is thought to confer some protection from this condition. The association between ε4 and AD is strongest when the patient has a positive family history of dementia. In addition, when two copies of ε4 are present, the association is further strengthened. The ε4/ε4 genotype occurs in only 1% of the normal population and in 19% of the familial AD population.
Relevance to psychiatry and behavioral science	ApoE testing can help to increase the specificity of diagnosis in a patient with a presentation that meets the clinical criteria for AD, but it does not predict whether the disease will develop in an asymptomatic individual. In a patient with the clinical diagnosis of AD, the presence of the ε4/ε4 genotype increases the probability that AD is the correct diagnosis to about 97%. On the other hand, approximately 42% of patients with AD do not have an ε4 allele. The test, therefore, is used in a specific context and not for screening or in the early stages of the diagnostic evaluation for dementia.
Preparation of patient	Patient counseling is mandatory. The patient's expectations, the value of a positive or a negative test, out-of-pocket costs, and implications for blood relatives as well as potential for discrimination in employment, insurability, or educational opportunities, should be discussed. A plan for a follow-up discussion of test results should be made.
Indications	• Increase specificity of diagnosis in the patient whose presentation meets the clinical criteria for AD • Not useful for presymptomatic testing
Reference range	No ε4 allele present Possible genotypes: ε3/ε3; ε3/ε2; ε2/ε2
Critical value(s)	None
Abnormal test	Genotypes: ε4/ε4; ε4/ε3; ε4/ε2
Interfering factors	None
Cross-references	None

McConnell LM, Sanders GD, Owens DK: Evaluation of genetic tests: APOE genotyping for the diagnosis of Alzheimer disease. Genet Test 3(1):47–53, 1999

Petersen RC, Waring SC, Smith GE, et al: Predictive value of APOE genotyping in incipient Alzheimer's disease. Ann NY Acad Sci 802:58–69, 1996

Aspartate transaminase (AST)	
Type of test	Blood
Explanation of test	AST is an enzyme found in liver cells and other metabolically active tissues, including the heart, muscle, kidney, and brain. AST levels rise with cellular injury. AST is used with other liver enzyme tests such as alanine transaminase (ALT) and alkaline phosphatase to evaluate liver function and detect liver damage. The pattern and degree of abnormality in each of these tests can be helpful in determining etiology. Extreme elevations in AST (>10 times the upper limit of normal [ULN]) are consistent with acute hepatitis, often of viral origin. As with ALT, the AST level in this condition can remain high for as long as 6 months. In chronic hepatitis, on the other hand, AST levels may be only minimally elevated (<4× ULN) or even high-normal. In liver disease such as cirrhosis, cancer, or biliary obstruction, AST levels may be nearly normal, but they are elevated more often than ALT. In liver damage due to alcohol, AST is usually significantly more elevated than ALT, a pattern unlike that seen in other causes of liver injury. In severe cirrhosis, the paradoxical finding of low AST may be seen, attributed to the loss of hepatocyte mass, with little remaining enzyme. In extrahepatic biliary obstruction, AST elevation is not as high as that of ALT. Although AST does increase in response to muscle or heart injury, creatine kinase or troponins are used instead in the workup of these conditions. The most common cause of mild AST elevation in the Western Hemisphere is nonalcoholic fatty liver disease.
Relevance to psychiatry and behavioral science	AST is one of the tests of liver health (liver "function") that is closely monitored in psychiatric practice, mainly because of the potential hepatotoxicity of psychotropic drugs. AST is also monitored in patients with alcoholism, substance-induced liver disease, and hepatitis. Elevation of AST may be found on routine screening. • If the patient has no clinical symptoms and no risk factors for liver disease, and AST is <3× ULN, a recheck is indicated after 1–3 months. • If the elevation persists, further investigation is needed. • If AST is >3× ULN on a single measurement, further investigation is needed. Elevation of AST may occur with initiation of a new psychotropic medication. In most cases, the AST increase is benign, and the lab value will revert to baseline within weeks of dose stabilization. Further investigation is needed in cases where the value does not normalize, or when alkaline phosphatase or bilirubin is also elevated.

Aspartate transaminase (AST) *(continued)*

Relevance to psychiatry and behavioral science *(continued)*	Pathological elevation of AST may occur with alcoholism, substance-induced liver disease, and hepatitis. It is important not to be misled by a normal AST value in a patient with established cirrhosis. In the patient with cirrhosis due to hepatitis C with a normal AST result, active hepatitis may be present, such that the patient would benefit from antiviral therapy, beta-blockers to prevent variceal bleeding, and other treatments. AST and ALT levels may also be normal in patients with hemochromatosis, in patients on methotrexate, or after jejunoileal bypass surgery, despite advanced liver disease. In all cases, the patient's history should be taken into account, and an effort should be made to identify other evidence of liver disease.
Preparation of patient	None needed
Indications	• A component of the liver function test panel • A component of the comprehensive metabolic panel • Monitoring medication effects on the liver • Evaluating patients with clinical symptoms of liver disease such as jaundice, abdominal pain, ascites, nausea, vomiting, or darkening of the urine (bilirubinuria) • Distinguishing hemolytic jaundice from jaundice due to liver dysfunction • Evaluating patients with hepatitis exposure or symptoms of hepatitis • Evaluating patients with alcoholism or other substance abuse • Monitoring the effects of treatment for liver disease
Reference range	Males: 14–20 U/L (0.23–0.33 µkat/L) Females: 10–36 U/L (0.17–0.60 µkat/L)
Critical value(s)	>200 IU/L indicates acute hepatic injury
Increased levels	• Active cirrhosis (alcohol or drug induced) • Hepatitis, acute and chronic • Infectious mononucleosis • Hepatic necrosis • Primary or metastatic carcinoma • Reye syndrome • Myocardial infarction (AST increase parallels that of creatine kinase)

Aspartate transaminase (AST) *(continued)*

Increased levels *(continued)*	• Numerous other conditions, including hypothyroidism, muscle trauma, muscle inflammation, toxic shock syndrome, cardiac catheterization, recent brain trauma, stroke, surgery, muscular dystrophy, pulmonary embolus, malignant hyperthermia, shock, exhaustion, and heat stroke • Drugs that are metabolized in the liver, including most psychotropics
Decreased levels	• Uremia in kidney failure • Chronic dialysis • Vitamin B_6 (pyridoxine) deficiency • Pregnancy • *Drugs:* vitamin C, ibuprofen, naltrexone, pindolol, and trifluoperazine
Interfering factors	Diabetic ketoacidosis, severe liver disease, uremia, and sample hemolysis may give spurious results.
Cross-references	Alcohol Use Disorder (Alcoholism) Alanine Transaminase (ALT) Hepatitis (Viral) Liver Function Tests (LFTs)

Gopal DV, Rosen HR: Abnormal findings on liver function tests: interpreting results to narrow the diagnosis and establish a prognosis. Postgrad Med 107:100–102, 105–109, 113–114, 2000

Theal RM, Scott K: Evaluating asymptomatic patients with abnormal liver function test results. Am Fam Physician 53(6):2111–2119, 1996

Basic metabolic panel (BMP)	
Type of test	Blood
Explanation of test	The basic metabolic panel includes the following eight tests: • Glucose • Calcium • Sodium • Potassium • Carbon dioxide • Chloride • Blood urea nitrogen (BUN) • Creatinine
Relevance to psychiatry and behavioral science	Although the BMP is often used in the emergency department (ED) setting as a means of rapid assessment of metabolic status, it is not the panel of choice for most patients with psychiatric presentations. In these cases, when general laboratory testing is considered necessary, the panel of choice would be the comprehensive metabolic panel, which includes liver function tests.
Preparation of patient	Ideally, the patient should be fasting overnight before testing, although this is rarely done. Mineral-containing supplements should be held for 12 hours before testing, and vigorous exercise should be avoided.
Indications	• Rapid workup in the ED setting • Monitoring specific lab values in the hospitalized patient
Reference range	See entries for individual tests.
Critical value(s)	
Increased levels	
Decreased levels	
Interfering factors	
Cross-references	Comprehensive Metabolic Panel (CMP) See entries for individual tests.

Bilirubin	
Type of test	Blood
Explanation of test	When red blood cells (RBCs) degrade, the hemoglobin component is broken down into unconjugated ("indirect") bilirubin. This form of bilirubin is transformed in the liver to conjugated ("direct") bilirubin, which is excreted into the gastrointestinal tract, where it is reduced by bacteria to urobilinogen. This compound may be excreted in feces or reabsorbed, in the latter case reappearing in urine or bile. These processes are shown in Figure 4 (see Appendix). When bilirubin levels are high, the patient may appear jaundiced. High levels may be a consequence of overproduction (usually due to hemolysis) or underexcretion (due to liver or biliary tract disease). A routine bilirubin test measures total bilirubin; if this is not elevated, no further testing is needed. If total bilirubin is elevated, the sample is fractionated to determine the percent conjugated versus unconjugated. *Conjugated Hyperbilirubinemia* When 30% or more of the bilirubin in a sample is in the conjugated (direct) form, conjugated hyperbilirubinemia exists; the differential diagnosis for this condition is shown in the "Increased Levels" section below. Any degree of bilirubinuria confirms the presence of conjugated hyperbilirubinemia. Other liver function test abnormalities are usually seen with conjugated hyperbilirubinemia. Patients with conjugated hyperbilirubinemia should be evaluated for hepatobiliary disease. *Unconjugated Hyperbilirubinemia* Patients with unconjugated hyperbilirubinemia should be evaluated for causes of RBC destruction such as hemolytic anemia. Isolated elevation of unconjugated bilirubin levels is most often caused by Gilbert syndrome, a common and usually benign genetic polymorphism associated with reduced glucuronidation of bilirubin. Establishing this diagnosis avoids costly and unnecessary testing for patients with intermittent jaundice.
Relevance to psychiatry and behavioral science	Elevation of bilirubin may be found on routine screening. • If the total bilirubin is <1.5× the upper limit of normal (ULN), recheck in 1–3 months unless there is clinical suspicion of disease. • If the total bilirubin is >1.5× ULN, determine the percentage that is unconjugated. If >70%, the diagnosis is probably Gilbert syndrome. If not, further investigation is needed.

Bilirubin *(continued)*	
Relevance to psychiatry and behavioral science *(continued)*	• If total bilirubin is >3× ULN, consultation is indicated because clinical disease is probable. Bilirubin may be elevated in alcoholism, cirrhosis, pernicious anemia, and cancer of the head of the pancreas, and as a drug reaction (e.g., to chlorpromazine or other phenothiazines).
Preparation of patient	The patient should fast for 4 hours before the test and should refrain from eating yellow foods (carrots, yellow beans, yams, pumpkin) for 3–4 days before the test.
Indications	• A component of the comprehensive metabolic panel • Presence of jaundice • History of alcohol overconsumption • Exposure to hepatitis • Signs of liver injury (e.g., from drugs) • Signs of liver disease such as cirrhosis or hepatitis • Evidence of bile duct obstruction • Hemolytic anemia (e.g., sickle cell disease)
Reference range	*Adults* Total bilirubin 0.3–1.0 mg/dL (5–17 μmol/L) Conjugated (direct) bilirubin 0.0–0.2 mg/dL (0.0–3.4 μmol/L)
Critical value(s)	Adults: >12 mg/dL (>200 μmol/L)
Increased levels	*Elevation of total bilirubin* • Hepatocellular jaundice (viral hepatitis, cirrhosis, infectious mononucleosis, drug reactions) • Obstructive jaundice (gallstones, cancer) • Hemolytic jaundice (posttransfusion, pernicious anemia, sickle cell anemia, transfusion reactions, Crigler-Najjar syndrome) • Gilbert syndrome • Dubin-Johnson syndrome • Pulmonary embolism • Congestive heart failure (CHF)

Bilirubin *(continued)*	
Increased levels *(continued)*	*Elevation of unconjugated (indirect) bilirubin* • Hemolytic anemia due to large hematoma • Trauma with large hematoma • Hemorrhagic pulmonary infarcts • Crigler-Najjar syndrome • Gilbert syndrome *Elevation of conjugated (direct) bilirubin* • Blockage of liver or bile ducts • Cancer of the head of the pancreas • Gallstones • Hepatitis • Liver trauma • Cirrhosis • Long-term alcohol overconsumption • Drug reaction • Dubin-Johnson syndrome *Drugs:* alcohol, morphine, theophylline, ascorbic acid, aspirin, chlordiazepoxide, chlorpromazine, and other phenothiazines
Decreased levels	Not applicable
Interfering factors	Bilirubin levels are slightly higher in males than in females. African Americans tend to have lower bilirubin values. Strenuous exercise may increase bilirubin levels. Fractionation tends to be unreliable in mild hyperbilirubinemia using standard "diazo" methods; newer, more precise methods may be required in these cases.
Cross-references	Alcohol Use Disorder (Alcoholism) Hepatitis (Viral) Liver Function Tests (LFTs)

Gopal DV, Rosen HR: Abnormal findings on liver function tests: interpreting results to narrow the diagnosis and establish a prognosis. Postgrad Med 107:100–102, 105–109, 113–114, 2000

Johnston DE: Special considerations in interpreting liver function tests. Am Fam Physician 59(8):2223–2230, 1999

Blood alcohol level (BAL)

Type of test	Blood
Explanation of test	Alcohol is rapidly absorbed from the gastrointestinal tract when taken on an empty stomach, with peak levels reached within 1 hour of ingestion. A small amount of alcohol is exhaled from the lungs and excreted in urine, but most is metabolized by the liver to acetaldehyde (and eventually to carbon dioxide and water). The normal liver has the capacity to metabolize about 1 drink per hour (12 oz of beer or 4–5 oz of wine or 1–1.5 oz of hard liquor). When more than 1 drink per hour is consumed, the alcohol level in the circulation rises. In the measurement of BAL, different systems of measurement yielding different units give rise to some confusion as to the meanings of particular levels; see the "Reference Range" section below. In general, a level equivalent to 0.08% or above is consistent with legal intoxication in most jurisdictions.
Relevance to psychiatry and behavioral science	Psychiatrists may be consulted for the evaluation of patients in the emergency department who are intoxicated or withdrawing from alcohol, and familiarity with the BAL is critical in this context. Alcohol is also often involved in suicide attempts. BAL may be used to monitor patients in treatment for alcohol dependence.
Preparation of patient	None needed
Indications	• Diagnosing alcohol intoxication • Diagnosing alcohol withdrawal • Determining the cause of coma • Providing legal evidence in the case of a motor vehicle accident or other event that may be related to intoxication • Monitoring employees suspected of drinking on the job • Monitoring patients in treatment for alcohol dependence or abuse • Monitoring ethanol level in patients treated for methanol poisoning
Reference range	Negative: <10 mg/dL, <2.00 mmol/L, <0.010% Negative by U.S. Department of Transportation (DOT): <20 mg/dL, <4.35 mmol/L, <0.020% Positive by U.S. DOT: >40 mg/dL, >8.68 mmol/L, >0.040% Positive under state laws: >80 mg/dL, >17.4 mmol/L, ≥0.08%

Blood alcohol level (BAL) *(continued)*

Critical value(s)	A BAL of >300 mg/dL is consistent with severe alcohol toxicity and requires immediate treatment for overdose.
	A BAL of >400 mg/dL can be associated with a fatal outcome.
	Symptoms of alcohol intoxication in the presence of a low BAL may signal a risk of serious impending withdrawal.
Increased levels	At BALs of 50–100 mg/dL, slowing of reflexes and impaired visual acuity are reported.
	At BALs >100 mg/dL, central nervous system depression is reported.
Decreased levels	Not applicable
Interfering factors	Ingestion of other alcohols (e.g., isopropanol or methanol) can confound ethanol measurement.
Cross-reference	Alcohol Use Disorder (Alcoholism)

Galanter M, Kleber HD (eds): The American Psychiatric Publishing Textbook of Substance Abuse Treatment, 4th Edition. Washington, DC, American Psychiatric Publishing, 2008

Hales RE, Yudofsky SC, Gabbard GO (eds): The American Psychiatric Publishing Textbook of Psychiatry, 6th Edition. Washington, DC, American Psychiatric Publishing, 2014

Blood urea nitrogen (BUN)

Type of test	Blood
Explanation of test	Urea is produced in the liver as a product of protein metabolism. It then circulates in the bloodstream and is excreted by the kidneys. Disease of the liver can be reflected in a decreased BUN, and disease of the kidneys can be reflected in an increased BUN. The latter condition is known as *azotemia*, and in its more severe form with accumulation of other waste products, uremia. The principal use of the BUN assay is to assess renal function. The ratio of BUN to creatinine level is used in the evaluation of conditions that cause a reduction in blood flow to the kidneys.
Relevance to psychiatry and behavioral science	Elevation of the BUN level in renal failure is associated with a range of psychiatric signs and symptoms, from fatigue, lassitude, and somnolence, to acute confusional states and delirium. Seizures can occur. In chronic renal disease, the BUN level correlates more closely with uremic symptoms than does the creatinine level.
Preparation of patient	No fasting is necessary. Dietary history may be needed to evaluate recent protein intake.
Indications	• A component of metabolic panels (basic metabolic panel and comprehensive metabolic panel) • Evaluating renal function (with creatinine) • Monitoring adequacy of dialysis and other interventions for kidney disease
Reference range	Adults ≤60 years: 6–20 mg/dL (2.1–7.1 mmol/L) Adults >60 years: 8–23 mg/dL (2.9–8.2 mmol/L) Children: 5–18 mg/dL (1.8–6.4 mmol/L) BUN : creatinine ratio normally between 10:1 and 20:1
Critical value(s)	>100 mg/dL (>35 mmol/L) indicates severe impairment of renal function
Increased levels	• Renal disease (acute or chronic) • Renal injury • Decreased renal blood flow in the context of congestive heart failure (CHF), dehydration, shock, stress, burns, or acute myocardial infarction • Rapid protein breakdown in the context of fever, burns, or cancer • Urinary tract obstruction • Hemorrhage into the gastrointestinal tract

Blood urea nitrogen (BUN) *(continued)*	
Increased levels *(continued)*	• Diabetic ketoacidosis • Excessive protein intake • Anabolic steroid use • Drugs: allopurinol, aminoglycoside antibiotics, aspirin (high-dose), carbamazepine, cephalosporins, chloral hydrate, furosemide, propranolol, and many others The ratio of BUN to creatinine may be increased when renal blood flow is compromised, as with dehydration or CHF. Excessive protein intake and gastrointestinal bleeding are other causes of an increased ratio.
Decreased levels	• Hepatic failure • Malnutrition with low protein intake • Celiac disease with impaired absorption • Syndrome of inappropriate antidiuretic hormone secretion (SIADH) • Overhydration • Pregnancy (2nd and 3rd trimester) • *Drugs:* chloramphenicol, streptomycin The ratio of BUN to creatinine may also be decreased (<10:1) in liver disease or malnutrition.
Interfering factors	Low muscle mass results in a lower BUN level. Higher BUN levels are found in elderly adults and in men.
Cross-references	Basic Metabolic Panel (BMP) Comprehensive Metabolic Panel (CMP) Creatinine (Cr) Syndrome of Inappropriate Antidiuretic Hormone Secretion (SIADH)

Calcium (Ca⁺⁺)	
Type of test	Blood
Explanation of test	Calcium has essential roles in neurotransmission, cardiac function, muscle contraction, blood clotting, and bone formation. The calcium level is maintained within a physiological range through the actions of parathyroid hormone and vitamin D. Most calcium is stored in bones and teeth; 1% circulates in blood, half bound to albumin and half in the free or ionized form. When the albumin level drops, the total calcium level drops, but the concentration of free calcium is unaffected. For this reason, the total calcium value is corrected when the albumin level is low. The correction formula for total calcium is as follows: $$[4 \text{ g/dL} - \text{plasma albumin}] \times 0.8 + \text{total serum calcium}$$ Alternatively, free calcium can be measured directly, but in this case, the specimen requires special handling and expedited processing.
Relevance to psychiatry and behavioral science	A calcium level may be drawn in the course of routine health screening and in the workup of various psychiatric signs and symptoms. Abnormal calcium levels may be associated with irritability, anxiety, depression, fatigue, lethargy, weakness, apathy, loss of appetite, delirium, nausea, vomiting, constipation, polyuria, polydipsia, bone pain, cardiac toxicity (including QTc prolongation and dysrhythmias), seizures, and coma. In patients with eating disorders, low calcium levels can result from chronic laxative abuse. A number of psychotropic drugs affect calcium levels, as noted in the "Increased Levels" and "Decreased Levels" sections below.
Preparation of patient	Ideally, the patient should fast overnight before the test and should avoid calcium supplements for at least 12 hours. When blood is being drawn, application of the tourniquet should be brief.
Indications	• Total calcium is a component of routine blood screening, included in both the basic metabolic panel (BMP) and the comprehensive metabolic panel. Ionized calcium can be ordered with the BMP instead of total calcium—for the same cost—but the specimen requires special handling. • Evaluating parathyroid function • Evaluating renal function • Symptoms of hypocalcemia, including abdominal cramps or skeletal muscle cramps and paresthesias in hands, feet, and circumoral areas • Symptoms of hypercalcemia

Calcium (Ca⁺⁺) *(continued)*	
Indications *(continued)*	• Workup for kidney stones • Workup for Paget disease and other bone diseases • Calcium monitoring post–renal transplantation • Calcium monitoring in certain cancers (breast, lung, multiple myeloma, kidney, or head/neck) • Monitoring treatment for abnormal calcium levels
Reference range	*Total serum calcium* Adults <60 years: 8.6–10.0 mg/dL (2.15–2.50 mmol/L) Adults 60–90 years: 8.8–10.2 mg/dL (2.20–2.55 mmol/L) Adults >90 years: 8.2–9.6 mg/dL (2.05–2.40 mmol/L) *Ionized serum calcium* Adults: 4.64–5.28 mg/dL (1.16–1.32 mmol/L)
Critical value(s)	*Total serum calcium* <4.4 mg/dL (<1.1 mmol/L): tetany, seizures >13 mg/dL (>3.25 mmol/L): cardiac toxicity, dysrhythmias, coma *Ionized serum calcium* <2.0 mg/dL (<1.1 mmol/L): tetany, seizures >7.0 mg/dL (>1.75 mmol/L): coma
Increased levels	*Total calcium >12 mg/dL (>3 mmol/L)* • Hyperparathyroidism • Cancer (parathyroid hormone [PTH]–producing tumors) • Granulomatous disease (tuberculosis, sarcoidosis) • Prolonged immobilization with fracture (children) • Excessive vitamin D intake • Paget disease (with elevated alkaline phosphatase) *Drugs:* lithium, paroxetine, phenobarbital, and propranolol, among others Other diseases and drugs that can cause hypercalcemia, but rarely severely enough to be symptomatic, include thyrotoxicosis, milk-alkali syndrome, adrenocortical insufficiency, and thiazide diuretics.

Calcium (Ca^{++}) *(continued)*	
Increased levels *(continued)*	*Increased ionized calcium* • Hyperparathyroidism • Cancer • PTH-producing tumors • Excessive vitamin D intake
Decreased levels	*Total calcium <4.0 mg/dL (<1.0 mmol/L)* • Hypoalbuminemia (pseudohypocalcemia, in which total calcium is affected; see correction formula in the "Explanation of Test" section above) • Hypoparathyroidism • Increased phosphorus level due to laxative abuse, renal failure, or cytotoxic drugs • Acute pancreatitis • Renal failure • Malabsorption due to gastrointestinal tract disease • Malnutrition, extreme dietary deficiency • Severe osteomalacia • Vitamin D deficiency, rickets • Magnesium deficiency • Alkalosis • Alcoholism, cirrhosis • Heritable resistance to PTH *Drugs:* carbamazepine, paroxetine, phenobarbital, and phenytoin, among others *Decreased ionized calcium* • Hyperventilation to treat increased intracranial pressure (total calcium may be normal) • Bicarbonate administration to treat metabolic acidosis • Hypoparathyroidism • Acute pancreatitis • Vitamin D or magnesium deficiency • Toxic shock syndrome • Syndrome of multiple organ failure

Calcium (Ca⁺⁺) *(continued)*	
Interfering factors	Normal values vary slightly with age (newborns vs. children vs. adults). Elevated serum protein increases total calcium level, whereas low serum protein decreases total calcium level. Abnormal levels of magnesium and phosphate affect calcium levels.
Cross-references	Anxiety Disorder (Secondary)
	Delirium
	Psychotic Disorder Due to Another Medical Condition

Carbamazepine level

Type of test	Blood
Explanation of test	Carbamazepine is an antiepileptic drug used to control complex partial seizures (formerly known as temporal lobe epilepsy) and generalized tonic-clonic seizures. It is also used to treat trigeminal neuralgia and other neuropathic pain syndromes.
Relevance to psychiatry and behavioral science	In neuropsychiatry, carbamazepine is used for the treatment of bipolar disorder, aggression, agitation in the context of dementia and traumatic brain injury; mood stabilization in patients with personality disorders; and as adjunctive treatment for patients with depression, schizophrenia, and schizoaffective disorder. For patients of Asian descent with the HLA-B*1502 genotype, carbamazepine should be used with extreme caution or avoided because of the risk of delayed hypersensitivity reactions (Stevens-Johnson syndrome and toxic epidermal necrolysis).
Preparation of patient	The patient should be instructed to hold the dose of medication until blood is drawn for testing. A trough level is checked, just before the morning dose.
Indications	• Routine monitoring of therapy. • Signs and symptoms of toxicity
Reference range	The reference ranges below have been established for seizures, but they do not necessarily apply to psychiatric indications. Levels should be at the lower end of the range if other antiepileptic drugs are used in combination. Total carbamazepine 4–12 μg/mL Free carbamazepine 1–3 μg/mL
Critical value(s)	Total carbamazepine ≥15 μg/mL Free carbamazepine ≥4 μg/mL
Increased levels	• Renal failure increases the level of the 10,11 epoxide • *Drugs:* calcium channel blockers, cimetidine, erythromycin, fluoxetine, influenza vaccine, isoniazid (INH), propoxyphene, verapamil, and vigabatrin
Decreased levels	• Noncompliance • *Drugs:* phenobarbital, primidone, and phenytoin
Interfering factors	None
Cross-reference	Manic Episode

Carbohydrate-deficient transferrin (CDT or %CDT)	
Type of test	Blood
Explanation of test	Transferrin is a protein that transports iron through the circulation to the bone marrow, where red blood cells are produced. Several forms of transferrin exist, with differing numbers of residues of the carbohydrate sialic acid attached. In normal individuals, each transferrin molecule has four sialic acid chains attached. In people who drink significant amounts of alcohol (>4 or 5 drinks daily for several weeks or more), the number of transferrin molecules with only one, two, or three sialic residues is increased. These molecules are referred to as *carbohydrate deficient*. These deficient transferrins can be measured in the blood and—along with aspartate transaminase, alanine transaminase, and gamma-glutamyltransferase values—provide a useful indicator of recent drinking. Some studies have shown this test to be positive in people drinking 60 g or more of ethanol daily for a minimum of 3 weeks. In general, the specificity of this test is high (97%) and the sensitivity is variable (65%–95%). With abstinence, the CDT value normalizes; the abnormal transferrin has a half-life of only 14–17 days.
Relevance to psychiatry and behavioral science	This is a useful test to supplement other measures in the evaluation of drinking behavior when the patient has not admitted that there is a problem. It can also be used to detect relapse in patients under treatment for alcohol dependence. In the latter case, the patient's own serial CDT values can provide a sensitive indicator of change in drinking status.
Preparation of patient	None needed
Indications	Detection of recent heavy alcohol consumption
Reference range	≤2.5%
Critical value(s)	≥2.6% or ≥26 IU/L suggests active drinking
Increased levels	• Recent heavy drinking • Genetic D variant of transferrin • Glycoprotein disorders • Primary biliary cirrhosis • Chronic active hepatitis
Decreased levels	Not applicable

Carbohydrate-deficient transferrin (CDT or %CDT) *(continued)*

Interfering factors	Differences in testing methods render %CDT results from some laboratories unreliable. Most of the reported research has been done with one of two assays: the Bio-Rad %CDT or the Kabi Pharmacia CDTect.
Cross-reference	Alcohol Use Disorder (Alcoholism)

Chrostek L, Cylwik B, Szmitkowski M, et al: The diagnostic accuracy of carbohydrate-deficient transferrin, sialic acid and commonly used markers of alcohol abuse during abstinence. Clin Chim Acta 364(1–2):167–171, 2006

Rinck D, Frieling H, Freitag A, et al: Combinations of carbohydrate-deficient transferrin, mean corpuscular erythrocyte volume, gamma-glutamyltransferase, homocysteine and folate increase the significance of biological markers in alcohol dependent patients. Drug Alcohol Depend 89(1):60–65, 2007

Carbon dioxide (CO_2)	
Type of test	Blood
Explanation of test	Although CO_2 exists in the body as a dissolved gas and as an ion, more than 95% of the total CO_2 content in normal plasma comes from the bicarbonate ion, which is regulated by the kidneys. Only a small fraction of total CO_2 content is contributed by dissolved CO_2 gas, which is regulated by the lungs. The total CO_2 (bicarbonate, carbonic acid, and other forms) provides a measure of the buffering capacity of the blood.
Relevance to psychiatry and behavioral science	This lab result may provide a clue to the presence of purging behaviors in patients with eating disorders. In addition, it may be increased in alcoholism and decreased in alcoholic ketosis, dehydration, head injury, or liver disease.
Preparation of patient	None needed
Indications	• A component of a blood panel for routine screening purposes • Used with blood gas values to determine whether an acid-base imbalance is primarily respiratory or metabolic in origin • Signs/symptoms of fluid/electrolyte imbalance • Monitoring chronic kidney disease
Reference range	Adults ≤60 years: 23–29 mEq/L (23–29 mmol/L) Adults >60 years: 23–31 mEq/L (23–31 mmol/L) Adults >90 years: 20–29 mEq/L (20–29 mmol/L)
Critical value(s)	<6.0 mEq/L
Increased levels	• Recurrent vomiting • Chronic obstructive pulmonary disease (emphysema) • Aldosteronism • *Drugs:* fludrocortisone, barbiturates, bicarbonates, hydrocortisone, loop diuretics, and steroids
Decreased levels	• Recurrent diarrhea • Acute renal failure • Starvation • Metabolic acidosis • Diabetic ketoacidosis • Addison disease • Salicylate overdose

Carbon dioxide (CO_2) *(continued)*	
Decreased levels *(continued)*	• Use of chlorothiazide diuretics • Poisoning with ethylene glycol or methanol • *Drugs:* methicillin, nitrofurantoin, tetracycline, thiazide diuretics, and triamterene
Interfering factors	None
Cross-references	Anorexia Nervosa Diabetes Mellitus Eating Disorders

Chest X ray (CXR)

Type of test	Imaging
Explanation of test	Routine CXR consists of two views: posteroanterior and left lateral. Upright films are preferred because supine films do not show fluid levels. Each film is taken at full inspiration. The entire procedure takes only a few minutes. Exposure to radiation is minimal unless the procedure is often repeated.
Relevance to psychiatry and behavioral science	Many of the conditions that can be diagnosed by CXR have an association with delirium. In the case of chronic conditions such as tuberculosis, depression may be prominent. In acute exacerbations of chronic obstructive pulmonary disease (COPD), anxiety may be the most pressing psychiatric symptom. Chronic changes consistent with emphysema are common among psychiatric patients, in large part because of the prevalence of smoking. Aspiration pneumonia is common among patients with dementia, particularly in later stages.
Preparation of patient	Clothing and jewelry covering the chest are removed. The patient wears a hospital gown. The female patient will be asked about pregnancy. The thyroid gland may be covered with a lead shield.
Indications	<ul><li>Delirium of unexplained etiology in an elderly patient</li><li>Dyspnea</li><li>Acute respiratory illness in any of the following patients:<ul><li>HIV positive</li><li>Over 40 years</li><li>Under 40 years with positive physical exam</li><li>Dementia</li><li>Patient with suspected severe acute respiratory syndrome (SARS) or anthrax</li><li>Febrile, neutropenic</li><li>Acute asthma with suspected pneumonia or pneumothorax</li><li>Acute COPD exacerbation with one or more of the following: leukocytosis, pain, history of coronary artery disease, or history of congestive heart failure (CHF)</li></ul></li></ul>
Abnormal findings	Foreign body, pneumonia, CHF, emphysema, abscess, cysts, pneumothorax, pleural effusion, tuberculosis, sarcoidosis, coccidioidomycosis, asbestosis, pulmonary embolus. May also detect bony abnormalities such as scoliosis, osteomyelitis, or osteoporosis.

Chest X ray (CXR) *(continued)*

Interfering factors	Conditions that interfere with the patient's ability to achieve full inspiration interfere with a complete exam. These include obesity, pain, CHF, and restrictive lung disease. In addition, if the patient is unable to travel to the radiology department, an anterior-to-posterior film will be obtained in bed in the upright position. This view is much less likely to reveal pathology, particularly in the area blocked by the heart.
Cross-references	Delirium
	Tuberculosis (TB)

Chlordiazepoxide level

Type of test	Blood
Explanation of test	Benzodiazepines are Schedule IV sedative-hypnotic drugs used to treat anxiety and insomnia. Chlordiazepoxide is also commonly used to treat alcohol withdrawal. This drug is an intermediate-acting benzodiazepine with a long half-life, with an active metabolite (nordiazepam). In general, levels of the parent drug and this metabolite are checked when either overdose or noncompliance is suspected or to detect use without a prescription. In the latter case, a urine drug screen would more likely be used and would detect the metabolite oxazepam.
Relevance to psychiatry and behavioral science	Toxicity with chronic benzodiazepine ingestion may manifest as confusion, disorientation, memory impairment, ataxia, decreased reflexes, and dysarthria. With acute overdose, the patient may exhibit somnolence, confusion, ataxia, decreased reflexes, vertigo, dysarthria, respiratory depression, and coma. More serious consequences usually involve co-ingestion of alcohol or other sedatives. If the ingestion was within 4 hours or if the patient is symptomatic, activated charcoal should be given and then repeated as these drugs undergo hepatic recirculation. Administration of flumazenil does not affect drug level but can result in symptomatic improvement.
Preparation of patient	None needed
Indications	• Screening for drug use • Suspicion of overdose • Signs of toxicity in a treated patient • Suspected noncompliance with prescribed therapy
Reference range	0.5–3.0 µg/mL
Critical value(s)	>5 µg/mL
Increased levels	• Overdose • Overuse • Poor metabolism • Hepatic encephalopathy
Decreased levels	Noncompliance
Interfering factors	None
Cross-references	Benzodiazepines Drug Screen (Toxicology Screen)

Chloride (Cl⁻)	
Type of test	Blood
Explanation of test	Chloride is an anion found in high concentration in the extracellular fluid, where it works to maintain osmotic pressure and water balance and acts as a buffer to maintain acid-base balance. Usually, chloride concentration rises and falls with sodium. However, the chloride level can change independently when an acid-base imbalance occurs, as the ion moves into and out of cells to maintain electrical neutrality. Chloride is ingested in food and table salt, with most absorbed in the gastrointestinal tract and the excess excreted in urine. Normally, blood levels are stable, with a slight decrease after meals when the stomach produces acid to aid digestion, using chloride from blood. When a massive diuresis occurs (such as with diabetes insipidus), chloride is lost through the urinary system. With significant vomiting or diarrhea, chloride is lost from the gastrointestinal tract. Chloride is measured as a routine component of electrolyte panels because it is useful in the diagnosis of acid-base and water balance problems. The results of the blood test may be followed up with a blood gas, urine chloride testing, or blood or urine sodium measurement.
Relevance to psychiatry and behavioral science	Chloride levels are affected by any process that involves loss of fluid from the gastrointestinal tract, change in acid-base balance, or change in sodium concentration. Neuropsychiatric conditions that may be associated with chloride derangements include diabetes insipidus, lithium intoxication, the syndrome of inappropriate antidiuretic hormone secretion (SIADH), polydipsia, porphyria, traumatic brain injury, eating disorders with purging behaviors, and hyperventilation.
Preparation of patient	The patient should fast for at least 8 hours before the test.
Indications	• A routine component of blood panels (including the electrolyte panel, basic metabolic panel, and comprehensive metabolic panel) • Suspicion of acidosis or alkalosis • Respiratory distress • Prolonged vomiting or diarrhea • Massive diuresis
Reference range	96–106 mEq/L (96–106 mmol/L) Values may be higher in patients >90 years.
Critical value(s)	<70 mEq/L or >120 mEq/L (<70 mmol/L or >120 mmol/L)

Chloride (Cl⁻) *(continued)*	
Increased levels	• Dehydration • Cushing syndrome (with high sodium level) • Metabolic acidosis (with prolonged diarrhea) • Respiratory alkalosis (with hyperventilation) • Primary hyperparathyroidism • Certain kidney diseases (e.g., renal tubular acidosis) • Diabetes insipidus • Salicylate intoxication • Traumatic brain injury with hypothalamic injury • Eclampsia • Excessive IV saline infusion • Drugs that increase sodium
Decreased levels	• Prolonged vomiting • Gastric suction • Salt-wasting diseases (e.g., SIADH, nephritis) • Chronic respiratory acidosis (e.g., in chronic obstructive pulmonary disease) • Burns • Metabolic alkalosis • Overhydration or water intoxication • Addison disease • Congestive heart failure • Acute intermittent porphyria • Ingestion of large amounts of antacids or baking soda • Drugs that decrease sodium
Interfering factors	Medications containing bromide can produce a positive reaction with some ion-selective electrode assays for chloride.
Cross-references	Eating Disorders Lithium Polydipsia (Psychogenic) Syndrome of Inappropriate Antidiuretic Hormone Secretion (SIADH)

Germon K: Fluid and electrolyte problems associated with diabetes insipidus and syndrome of inappropriate antidiuretic hormone. Nurs Clin North Am 22:785–796, 1987

Siragy HM: Hyponatremia, fluid-electrolyte disorders, and the syndrome of inappropriate antidiuretic hormone secretion: diagnosis and treatment options. Endocr Pract 12:446–457, 2006

Clonazepam level

Type of test	Blood
Explanation of test	Benzodiazepines are Schedule IV sedative-hypnotic drugs used to treat anxiety and insomnia. Clonazepam is an intermediate-acting drug with a long half-life. In general, levels are checked when either overdose or noncompliance is suspected, or to detect use without a prescription. For the latter indication, a urine drug screen would more likely be used than a blood level.
Relevance to psychiatry and behavioral science	Toxicity with chronic benzodiazepine ingestion may manifest as confusion, disorientation, memory impairment, ataxia, decreased reflexes, and dysarthria. There is some evidence that use of long-acting benzodiazepines such as clonazepam is associated with an increased risk of motor vehicle accidents and falls in elderly patients, even when levels are in the therapeutic range. With acute benzodiazepine overdose, patients may exhibit somnolence, confusion, ataxia, decreased reflexes, vertigo, dysarthria, respiratory depression, and coma. More serious consequences usually involve co-ingestion of alcohol or other sedatives. If the ingestion was within 4 hours or if the patient is symptomatic, activated charcoal should be given and then repeated, because these drugs undergo hepatic recirculation. Administration of flumazenil does not affect drug level but can result in symptomatic improvement.
Preparation of patient	None needed
Indications	• Screening for drug use • Suspicion of overdose • Signs of toxicity in a treated patient • Suspected noncompliance with prescribed therapy
Reference range	10–75 ng/mL (for dosages up to 6 mg daily)
Critical value(s)	>100 ng/mL
Increased levels	• Overdose • Overuse • Poor metabolism • Hepatic encephalopathy
Decreased levels	Noncompliance
Interfering factors	None
Cross-references	Benzodiazepines Drug Screen (Toxicology Screen)

Clozapine level	
Type of test	Blood
Explanation of test	A therapeutic range is not well established. There is some evidence that 100 ng/mL is the minimum possible therapeutic level. Some sources suggest the reference range noted below. For treatment-refractory schizophrenia, the recommended lower limit of the reference range is 350 ng/mL.
Relevance to psychiatry and behavioral science	Clozapine is the prototype atypical antipsychotic drug— the first to be marketed and still widely considered the most efficacious. Use of clozapine is limited by its potential to cause agranulocytosis and other serious adverse effects. It is used primarily to treat schizophrenia in cases where other drugs have proven ineffective, particularly to reduce suicidality in this population. It is also used in the treatment of bipolar disorder, Parkinson's disease with psychosis, dementia with Lewy bodies, and psychosis in patients with tardive dyskinesia.
Preparation of patient	None needed
Indications	• Suspected noncompliance • Signs/symptoms of toxicity • Poor response to treatment

Reference range	See notes above in "Explanation of Test"
	
	200–700 ng/mL
	
	This reference range applies to treatment of major psychiatric disorders such as schizophrenia but not to the treatment of psychosis arising in the context of medical conditions such as Parkinson's disease. In the latter cases, lower blood levels may be clinically effective.
	
	For treatment-refractory schizophrenia:
	    clozapine: >350 ng/mL
	    clozapine + norclozapine: >450 ng/mL

Critical value(s)	>1,200 ng/mL
Increased levels	Toxicity
Decreased levels	Treatment nonresponse Noncompliance
Interfering factors	None
Cross-reference	Clozapine in "Psychotropic Medications" section

Complete blood count (CBC)	
Type of test	Blood
Explanation of test	The CBC is an automated count of blood cells that reports the following information: white blood cell (WBC), red blood cell (RBC), and platelet counts per volume; platelet volume; hemoglobin content; hematocrit; and red cell indices (mean corpuscular volume [MCV], mean corpuscular hemoglobin [MCH], mean corpuscular hemoglobin concentration [MCHC], and red cell distribution of width [RDW]).
	MCH is a calculation of the average amount of oxygen-carrying hemoglobin in the RBCs. Macrocytic RBCs have higher MCH values, and microcytic RBCs have lower MCH values. MCHC is a calculation of the average concentration of hemoglobin in the RBCs. Low MCHC, or hypochromia, is seen with diseases such as iron deficiency anemia or thalassemia, when hemoglobin is diluted. High MCHC, or hyperchromia, is seen with conditions such as burns, where hemoglobin is concentrated.
	RDW is a calculation of the variance in size (anisocytosis) and shape (poikilocytosis) of RBCs.
	If a *differential* is ordered with the CBC, types of WBCs are identified either manually or by automated means, and the percentage of each type is reported.
	Unusual cell types or morphology may be noted on examination of the blood smear and reported with the routine CBC.
Relevance to psychiatry and behavioral science	This is an important basic screening test that should be familiar to all psychiatrists. It aids in the diagnosis of many medical conditions that can cause symptoms reminiscent of primary psychiatric diseases. The CBC is a high-yield, low-cost test.
Preparation of patient	Fasting is not required. Physiological stress should be avoided just prior to the test.
Indications	• A basic screening panel for hospital admission and general health status • Presurgical evaluation • Monitoring after surgery • Clinical signs/symptoms such as fever, fatigue, weakness, or abnormal bleeding or bruising • Clinical suspicion of infection or inflammation

Complete blood count (CBC) *(continued)*

Reference range	*Adults*
	
	    MCH 28–34 pg/cell
	
	    MCHC 32–36 g/dL
	
	    RDW 11.5%–14.5%
	
	For other values, see individual test components.

Critical value(s)	See entries for test components.
Increased levels	
Decreased levels	
Interfering factors	
Cross-references	Mean Corpuscular Volume (MCV) Red Blood Cell Count (RBC) White Blood Cell Count (WBC)

Comprehensive metabolic panel (CMP)

Type of test	Blood
Explanation of test	The CMP includes the following 14 tests: • Glucose • Calcium • Albumin • Protein (total protein) • Sodium • Potassium • Carbon dioxide • Chloride • Blood urea nitrogen (BUN) • Creatinine • Alanine transaminase (ALT) • Aspartate transaminase (AST) • Bilirubin • Alkaline phosphatase
Relevance to psychiatry and behavioral science	In patients presenting with psychiatric signs/symptoms, the CMP may be useful for rapid assessment of metabolic status. In psychiatry and behavioral medicine, this panel is used in preference to the basic metabolic panel because it includes liver function tests. The CMP is a high-yield, low-cost test.
Preparation of patient	Usually none, although overnight fasting yields a more meaningful glucose measurement in many cases.
Indications	• Metabolic screen for patients presenting with psychiatric signs/symptoms • Routine health screen • Monitoring of specific lab values in the hospitalized patient
Reference range	See entries for individual tests.
Critical value(s)	
Increased levels	
Decreased levels	
Interfering factors	
Cross-references	Basic Metabolic Panel (BMP) See entries for individual tests.

Cranial computed tomography (head CT or CAT scan)	
Type of test	Imaging
Explanation of test	Computed tomography (CT) images are created by attenuation of X-ray beams by tissues of differing density. Brightness on the CT scan is proportional to the density of the tissue. Bone and calcium are very bright (white). Cerebrospinal fluid and fat are black. Gray matter is lighter gray than white matter. CT study can be performed nonenhanced ("without" contrast), or it can be enhanced with iodinated dye administered intravenously ("with" contrast). Contrast improves visualization of lesions such as stroke, tumor, and abscess. Certain brain structures are normally enhanced with intravenous contrast dye. When a head CT is ordered, the "brain window" is the standard one used, but other windows can be specified for other purposes (e.g., bone window or subdural window). CT is preferred to magnetic resonance imaging (MRI) in the detection of calcified lesions, meningeal tumors, and acute blood. CT is less degraded by motion artifact than is MRI. It is inferior to MRI in the detection of ischemia or demyelination, and it is not as well able to visualize brain stem, cerebellum, or temporal lobes because of artifact created at the bone-tissue interface. Spatial resolution of structures is inferior to that of MRI. Even with thin slices, CT is a shorter study than MRI, and the cost is about half that of MRI. CT slice thickness ranges from 1 to 10 mm. Thicker cuts reduce the time of the study but also further reduce sensitivity because smaller lesions may be missed. The axial CT scan image is presented as though one were viewing the brain from the foot of the bed while the patient lies supine, so the right side of the brain appears on the viewer's left.
Relevance to psychiatry and behavioral science	CT is a relatively low-cost, high-yield testing modality in certain patient populations, including those with new-onset headaches, new neurological deficits, or acute head trauma. In addition, CT (or MRI) is indicated for patients with a first episode of psychosis, prolonged catatonia, or first onset after age 50 years of psychosis, mood disorder, or personality disorder.
Preparation of patient	The scan takes approximately 10 minutes. Radiation exposure is little more than that of plain films of the skull, but cumulative effects can be significant. *The CT contrast agent is more likely than MRI gadolinium to cause an allergic reaction, which can be serious.* Anaphylaxis can occur. Allergic reactions are more common in patients who are allergic to seafood or who have a history of asthma.

Cranial computed tomography (head CT or CAT scan) *(continued)*

Indications	• Sudden-onset severe or unilateral headache • Suspected carotid or vertebral dissection • Ipsilateral Horner syndrome • New headache in a pregnant patient (without contrast) • New headache with suspected meningitis or encephalitis (without contrast, to assess intracranial pressure increase) • Transient ischemic attack involving carotid or vertebro-basilar territories (combined with CT angiography) • New focal neurological deficit • Suspected subarachnoid hemorrhage (without contrast) • Brain parenchymal hemorrhage • Ataxia of acute onset • First episode of psychosis with atypical presentation • First onset of psychosis, mood disorder, or personality disorder after age 50 years • Prolonged catatonia
Normal test	• Normal anatomical landmarks identified • No midline shift • No extracerebral fluid accumulation (subdural or epidural) • No abnormal hypodense or hyperdense areas • If atrophy is present, it is generalized and mild, or moderate in a patient of advanced age. • A thick skull is usually a normal variant. • A marked hyperostosis of the frontal bone is common in older women without brain pathology.
Abnormal test	The following appear dark (less dense) on CT because of accumulation of extravascular fluid: • Infarction • Demyelination • Inflammation • Gliosis • Most cancers • Cysts

Cranial computed tomography (head CT or CAT scan) *(continued)*	
Abnormal test *(continued)*	The following appear light (more dense) on CT: • Acute blood • Meningiomas • Thrombosis • Calcified masses • Calcified tubers • Colloid cysts • Certain primary lymphomas
Interfering factors	Motion artifact interferes with image acquisition.
Cross-reference	Magnetic Resonance Imaging (MRI)

Holt RE: The role of computed tomography of the brain in psychiatry. Psychiatr Med 1(3):275–285, 1983

National Guideline Clearinghouse: ACR Appropriateness Criteria. Available at: http://www.ngc.gov. Accessed May 2010.

Creatine kinase (CK) (also known as creatine phosphokinase (CPK))	
Type of test	Blood
Explanation of test	CK is an enzyme involved in ATP (adenosine triphosphate) production and storage. It is found in the heart and skeletal muscles, and in smaller concentrations in brain tissue. Circulating CK is a marker of injury to these CK-rich tissues. Three isoforms of CK exist: • CK-BB (CK_1), localized mostly in brain (but also smooth muscle, thyroid gland, lungs, and prostate) • CK-MB (CK_2), localized mostly in cardiac muscle (but also tongue and diaphragm) • CK-MM (CK_3), localized mostly in skeletal muscle In the blood of healthy people, almost all CK is in the MM form. Elevation of CK-MM outside the normal range indicates skeletal muscle injury. CK-BB from the central nervous system (CNS) rarely enters the circulation; CNS injury may be reflected in only a slight elevation of total CK. Elevation of CK-MB suggests cardiac muscle injury and has traditionally been used to diagnose myocardial infarction (MI), using serial blood tests. It is important to note that although the absolute level of CK-MB may be elevated with exercise, intramuscular injection, stroke, seizure, pericarditis, pneumonia, pulmonary embolism, and other lung diseases, the relative percentage is not increased in these conditions as it is in acute MI.
Relevance to psychiatry and behavioral science	The two most important conditions in the differential diagnosis for the psychiatric patient with elevated total CK are acute MI (with elevated CK-MB in addition to CK-MM) and neuroleptic malignant syndrome (with elevated CK-MM). CK elevation may also be seen in patients with seizure, stroke, traumatic brain injury, delirium tremens, carbon monoxide poisoning, or dystonic reactions. CK (and CK-MM) elevation can be induced by interventions such as intramuscular injections, use of physical restraints, or electroconvulsive therapy (ECT). Atypical antipsychotics and haloperidol are associated with a variable elevation of CK-MM in the absence of muscle pathology in about 10% of treated patients. Although the elevation can be extreme, renal function is not impaired. It has been hypothesized that this antipsychotic-related CK elevation arises from a change in skeletal muscle cell permeability in susceptible individuals. This "asymptomatic elevation" is a diagnosis of exclusion.

Creatine kinase (CK) (also known as creatine phosphokinase (CPK)) *(continued)*	
Preparation of patient	If the test is performed to evaluate skeletal muscle injury, the patient should avoid strenuous physical activity for 24 hours.
Indications	• Diagnosing MI • Evaluating muscle injury in chronic muscular diseases such as muscular dystrophy • Evaluating muscle injury in acute or subacute conditions such as myositis • Detecting muscle injury from statins and other drugs, such as antipsychotic medications • Diagnosing CNS disorders such as Reye syndrome
Reference range	Males: 38–174 U/L (0.63–2.90 µkat/L) Females: 26–140 U/L (0.46–2.38 µkat/L) CK-MM 96%–100% of total CK-MB 0%–4% of total CK-BB 0%
Critical value(s)	None
Increased levels	*Total CK (and CK-MM)* • MI • Myocarditis • Cardioversion • Open heart surgery • Muscular dystrophy • Myositis • Stroke • Delirium tremens • ECT • Recent electric shock or electromyogram • Malignant hyperthermia • Neuroleptic malignant syndrome • Reye syndrome • Subarachnoid hemorrhage • Late pregnancy or childbirth • Hypothyroidism

Creatine kinase (CK)
(also known as creatine phosphokinase (CPK)) *(continued)*

Increased levels *(continued)*	*Total CK (and CK-MM)* (continued)
	• Acute psychosis
	• Acute mania
	• Traumatic brain injury
	• Cancer of prostate, bladder, or gastrointestinal tract
	• Cocaine intoxication with rhabdomyolysis
	• Eosinophilia-myalgia syndrome
	• Seizure
	CK-MB
	• MI
	• Duchenne muscular dystrophy
	• Subarachnoid hemorrhage
	• Reye syndrome
	• Surgery or muscle trauma
	• Circulatory failure or shock
	• Myocarditis
	• Chronic renal failure
	• Malignant hyperthermia
	• Hypothermia
	• Carbon monoxide poisoning
	• Polymyositis
	• Myoglobinemia
	• Rocky Mountain spotted fever
	CK-BB
	• Reye syndrome
	• Certain cancers
	• Severe shock
	• Neurosurgery
	• Traumatic brain injury
	• Hypothermia
	• After coronary bypass surgery
	• Newborns

Creatine kinase (CK) (also known as creatine phosphokinase (CPK)) *(continued)*	
Decreased levels	Not usually of diagnostic significance. Associated with bed rest, small muscle mass, or early pregnancy.
Interfering factors	Higher CK levels are seen in individuals with more muscle mass and in African Americans. Heavy exercise (e.g., weight lifting, contact sports, or prolonged exercise) elevates CK levels. Intramuscular injections and use of physical restraints elevate CK levels.
Cross-reference	Neuroleptic Malignant Syndrome (NMS)

Meltzer HY, Cola PA, Parsa M: Marked elevations of serum creatine kinase activity associated with antipsychotic drug treatment. Neuropsychopharmacology 15(4):395–405, 1996

Creatinine (Cr)

Type of test	Blood, 24-hour urine
Explanation of test	Creatinine is a waste product continually produced in skeletal muscle by the breakdown of creatine phosphate. The amount produced depends on the muscle mass of the individual. All creatinine that is filtered by the kidneys is eliminated, so the level of creatinine in the blood reflects the glomerular filtration rate (GFR). The serum creatinine level doubles when the GFR is reduced by 50%. Serum creatinine is used with blood urea nitrogen (BUN) to evaluate kidney function, with both elevated in kidney disease.

<table>
<tr>
<td></td>
<td>

Traditionally, creatinine clearance has been estimated by the Cockcroft-Gault formula:

Creatinine clearance (mL/min) = (140−age) × weight (kg) / 72 × serum creatinine (mg/dL).

For females, the result is multiplied by a correction factor of 0.85.

The newer and more accurate MDRD (Modification of Diet in Renal Disease Study) equation is now used by many laboratories, and an estimated GFR is reported along with serum creatinine. If this estimate is not provided, the GFR can be obtained by entering patient data (age, ethnicity, gender, and serum creatinine value) into a calculator such as that provided on the Web site www.mdcalc.com/mdrd-gfr-equation/.

The ratio of BUN to creatinine is sometimes helpful in determining what underlies an abnormal creatinine value. A normal ratio is between 10:1 and 20:1.

- An increased ratio suggests reduced blood flow to the kidney due to conditions such as congestive heart failure (CHF) or dehydration, or increased protein (urea nitrogen) from gastrointestinal bleeding or dietary sources.

- A decreased ratio suggests malnourishment or liver disease with decreased urea formation.

</td>
</tr>
</table>

Creatinine (Cr) *(continued)*

Relevance to psychiatry and behavioral science	Delirium is associated with various conditions in which creatinine levels are elevated, including acute renal failure (in which creatinine increase is proportional to BUN increase) and dehydration (in which creatinine increase is less than BUN increase). Creatinine is a component of the laboratory evaluation for newly hospitalized patients with suspected eating disorders. The level may be increased, or it may be normal despite significant renal dysfunction due to the confounding influence of decreased muscle mass. Lithium may cause true creatinine elevation, with compromise of renal function and reduced clearance of other drugs. Other psychotropic drugs may cause an elevation in creatinine that is without clinical significance.
Preparation of patient	None needed
Indications	• A component of the basic and comprehensive metabolic panels • Evaluating general health status • Suspicion of kidney disease or dysfunction • Monitoring known kidney disease • Monitoring renal function on nephrotoxic drugs (e.g., aminoglycosides) • Preoperative assessment • Preparing for administration of contrast agents for imaging
Reference range	*Adults 18–60 years* Males: 0.9–1.3 mg/dL (80–115 µmol/L) Females: 0.6–1.1 mg/dL (53–97 µmol/L) *Adults 61–90 years* Males: 0.8–1.3 mg/dL (71–115 µmol/L) Females: 0.6–1.2 mg/dL (53–106 µmol/L) *Adults >90 years* Males: 1.0–1.7 mg/dL (88–150 µmol/L) Females: 0.6–1.3 mg/dL (53–115 µmol/L)
Critical value(s)	10 mg/dL in a nondialysis patient
Increased levels	*Kidney diseases* • Glomerulonephritis • Pyelonephritis • Acute tubular dysfunction

Creatinine (Cr) *(continued)*	
Increased levels *(continued)*	*Kidney diseases (continued)* • Nephrotic syndrome • Interstitial nephritis • Amyloidosis *Other conditions* • Reduced blood flow to the kidney (atherosclerosis) • Urinary tract obstruction (kidney stone or prostate enlargement) • Dehydration • CHF • Shock • Hemorrhage • Muscle injury • Myasthenia gravis • Gigantism or acromegaly • High protein diet • Increased muscle mass *Drugs:* ACE inhibitors, angiotensin receptor blockers, gabapentin, lithium, and others
Decreased levels	• Pregnancy • Decreased muscle mass • Burns • Carbon monoxide poisoning
Interfering factors	Many drugs falsely elevate creatinine levels, including ascorbic acid, barbiturates, some cephalosporins, cimetidine, clonidine, levodopa, and trimethoprim-sulfamethoxazole. Creatine supplementation increases creatinine levels. Age is not a significant interfering factor in creatinine measurement, because muscle mass tends to decrease at the same time that renal function declines. The net effect involves only small changes in serum creatinine.
Cross-references	Blood Urea Nitrogen (BUN) Lithium

Levey AS, Bosch JP, Lewis JB, et al; Modification of Diet in Renal Disease Study Group: A more accurate method to estimate glomerular filtration rate from serum creatinine: a new prediction equation. Ann Intern Med 130(6):461–470, 1999

Cytochrome P450 (CYP450) genotyping: AmpliChip CYP450 test

Type of test	Genetic
Explanation of test	The Roche AmpliChip CYP450 Test provides genotyping for two CYP450 isoenzymes involved in drug metabolism: CYP2D6 and CYP2C19. The test classifies individuals into three C19 phenotypes (extensive, intermediate, and poor metabolizers) and four 2D6 phenotypes (ultra-rapid, extensive, intermediate, and poor metabolizers). The AmpliChip does not measure the CYP2C19*17 genotype, which is associated with ultra-rapid metabolism. Unlike most other genetic testing, which is developed by individual laboratories, the AmpliChip is a commercially developed kit used by a number of designated laboratories. When the kit was approved by the U.S. Food and Drug Administration, only the assay's technical performance was reviewed; neither clinical validity nor clinical utility was fully addressed. The Evaluation of Genomic Applications in Practice and Prevention (EGAPP) Working Group performed these analyses and published the following findings in 2007: 1) sensitivity and specificity of the test are high for common polymorphisms, but not as good for rarer polymorphisms or for gene deletions or duplications; 2) inadequate evidence is available to support the clinical validity of the test; and 3) no evidence exists to support clinical utility of the test.
Relevance to psychiatry and behavioral science	Psychotropic drugs metabolized by CYP2D6 include risperidone, venlafaxine, aripiprazole, duloxetine, and atomoxetine, among many others. The poor metabolizer phenotype occurs in 7% of Caucasians and 1%–3% of those in other ethnic groups. Poor metabolism at 2D6 is thought to underlie adverse effects of risperidone. Drugs metabolized by CYP2C19 include citalopram and tricyclic antidepressants. The poor metabolizer phenotype at 2C19 is found in 3%–4% of Caucasians and 14%–21% of people of Asian descent. Given these ethnic differences, it is not surprising that a great deal of interest was generated when the AmpliChip became available. Most attention was focused initially on the ability of the test to predict drug concentration (and response) for selective serotonin reuptake inhibitor (SSRI) antidepressants related to 2D6 isoenzyme polymorphism. At least in theory, individuals with more than two copies of the active ("wild type") alleles—ultra-rapid metabolizers—would have subtherapeutic drug concentrations at usual medication doses, those with two copies of active alleles—extensive metabolizers—would have expected drug concentrations, and those with two copies of inactive alleles—poor metabolizers—would have higher, potentially toxic drug concentrations at usual doses. The review conducted by the EGAPP Working Group found that the literature did support the idea that individuals with two inactive alleles had reduced metabolism, but the metabolic function of the other groups overlapped considerably. The EGAPP group discouraged use of CYP450 genotyping for patients starting SSRI treatment until further clinical trials were completed.

Cytochrome P450 (CYP450) genotyping: AmpliChip CYP450 test *(continued)*	
Preparation of patient	None needed
Indications	Clinical suspicion of poor metabolizer status in an SSRI-treated patient
Abnormal test	Report returned indicating that the patient is a poor metabolizer (two copies of inactive allele)
Normal test	Report returned indicating that the patient is an extensive metabolizer (two copies of active allele)
Interfering factors	None
Cross-references	None

de Leon J, Armstrong SC, Cozza KL: Clinical guidelines for psychiatrists for the use of pharmacogenetic testing for CYP450 2D6 and CYP450 2C19. Psychosomatics 47(1):75–85, 2006

Evaluation of Genomic Applications in Practice and Prevention (EGAPP) Working Group: Recommendations from the EGAPP Working Group: testing for cytochrome P450 polymorphisms in adults with nonpsychotic depression treated with selective serotonin reuptake inhibitors. Genet Med 9(12):819–825, 2007

Diazepam level	
Type of test	Blood
Explanation of test	Benzodiazepines are Schedule IV sedative-hypnotic drugs used to treat anxiety and insomnia. Diazepam is a highly lipophilic benzodiazepine with a short transit through the circulation before being deposited in fatty tissue, where it can accumulate. It is then released erratically back into the circulation. Both diazepam and its active metabolite nordiazepam have long elimination half-lives. Diazepam levels generally have little clinical significance, except when extremely high or low. Levels are rarely checked except to confirm overdose, noncompliance, or use without a prescription. In the latter case, a urine drug screen is more likely to be ordered than a blood level.
Relevance to psychiatry and behavioral science	Toxicity with chronic benzodiazepine ingestion may manifest as confusion, disorientation, memory impairment, ataxia, decreased reflexes, and dysarthria. With acute overdose, the patient may exhibit somnolence, confusion, ataxia, decreased reflexes, vertigo, dysarthria, respiratory depression, and coma. More serious consequences usually involve co-ingestion of alcohol or other sedatives. If the ingestion was within 4 hours or if the patient is symptomatic, activated charcoal should be given and then repeated, because these drugs undergo hepatic recirculation. Administration of flumazenil does not affect drug level.
Preparation of patient	None needed
Indications	• Screening for drug use • Suspicion of overdose • Signs of toxicity in a treated patient • Suspected noncompliance with prescribed therapy
Reference range	Diazepam 0.2–1.0 µg/mL Nordiazepam 0.06–1.80 µg/mL
Critical value(s)	Nordiazepam >2.50 µg/mL
Increased levels	• Overdose • Overuse • Poor metabolism • Hepatic encephalopathy
Decreased levels	Noncompliance
Interfering factors	None
Cross-references	Benzodiazepines Drug Screen (Toxicology Screen)

Drug screen (toxicology screen)	
Type of test	Urine
Explanation of test	The toxicology screening test for drugs of abuse is usually performed on a random urine sample for a selected panel of drugs. Different panels are available, depending on the lab (e.g., seven drugs with alcohol, seven drugs without alcohol). Positive results (above a predetermined cutoff value) may be followed up with more sensitive and specific testing that identifies the exact drug. The classes of drugs most often included in the screening panel include opioids, cocaine, amphetamines, barbiturates, benzodiazepines, phencyclidine (PCP), and cannabinoids (marijuana). As an alternative to the drug panel, tests may be ordered individually. Some drugs, including many currently abused "club drugs," are not included in many of the currently designed panels. These drugs include 3,4-methylenedioxymethamphetamine (MDMA; Ecstasy), oxycodone (OxyContin), and buprenorphine/naloxone (Suboxone). Others, such as gamma-hydroxybutyrate (GHB), have such a short half-life that detection would be difficult, even if they were included. Complicating the interpretation of opioid screening is the fact that some opioids are metabolized to other opioids, such that their presence may indicate metabolism rather than additional abuse. The following guidelines may be helpful in interpretation: • If free morphine as a percentage of free codeine is <55%, morphine may have come from metabolism of codeine. • Detection of 6-acetylmorphine with morphine is definitive evidence of heroin use, but this intermediate metabolite is short lived (<8 hours). • Failure to detect 6-acetylmorphine with morphine does not rule out heroin use, because the half-life of the metabolite is short. • If free hydromorphone as a percentage of hydrocodone is <30%, hydromorphone may have come from metabolism of hydrocodone. • If hydrocodone as a percentage of free codeine is <40%, hydrocodone may have come from metabolism of codeine. • If free hydromorphone as a percentage of free morphine is <25%, hydromorphone may have come from metabolism of morphine.

Drug screen (toxicology screen) *(continued)*

Explanation of test *(continued)*	For amphetamines, cocaine, and opioids, urine screening detects drug use in the past 2–3 days. For chronic cannabinoid use (marijuana and its metabolites), urine screening detects drug use in the last several weeks. For barbiturates, urine detection depends on the specific drug; short-acting barbiturates are detected in urine up to 24 hours, and long-acting barbiturates are detected in urine up to 3 weeks.
	For specific legal or employment purposes, other sampling methods may be used. Hair samples reflect drug use within the last 2–3 months. Saliva samples can detect drugs used in the previous 24 hours. Sweat samples can be collected over a period of days to weeks on an absorbent patch and can indicate drug use during that period. For alcohol screening, blood is most often used, as discussed in the Blood Alcohol Level (BAL) entry.
Relevance to psychiatry and behavioral science	Urine drug screening is commonly used in the emergency department (ED) setting. It is also used to monitor known substance abusers in treatment. It is used routinely in certain occupations, and it can be requested for legal purposes.
Preparation of patient	None needed
Indications	• Patient in the ED with unexplained symptoms • Patient in the ED after an accident, when alcohol or substance use is suspected • Patient suspected of drug use • Monitoring known drug users • Pregnant women at risk of drug use • Neonates with signs of drug intoxication
Reference range	Refer to lab documentation.
Critical value(s)	None
Positive test	Positive screening tests are confirmed by more sensitive and specific assays. Positive confirmation in the absence of confounding factors means that the patient has ingested the drug. In some cases, the window of time during which the drug was taken can be inferred.
Negative test	If the drug is not present or is present below the predetermined cutoff for a positive test, the report is returned as "not detected." As discussed above, a negative result does not necessarily mean that the drug was never taken; it may have been eliminated by the body by the time the test was taken, or it may have been present below the detection limit for the assay. It is also possible that the drug taken was not included in that drug screening panel.

Drug screen (toxicology screen) *(continued)*

Interfering factors	*Opioids:* False-positive results may occur with rifampin, fluoroquinolones, and unwashed poppy seeds.
	Amphetamines: False-positive results may occur with selegiline and Vicks inhalers (the latter at twice the recommended dosage).
	PCP: False-positive results may occur with venlafaxine overdose or dextromethorphan use.
	False-negative results may occur from dilute urine or may be due to rapid drug metabolism.
Cross-reference	Blood Alcohol Level (BAL)

Moeller KE, Lee KC, Kissack JC: Urine drug screening: practical guide for clinicians. Mayo Clin Proc 83(1):66–76, 2008

Reisfield GM, Bertholf RL: "Practical guide" to urine drug screening clarified. Mayo Clin Proc 83:848–849; author reply 849, 2008

Electrocardiogram (ECG or EKG)	
Type of test	Electrophysiology
Explanation of test	The ECG records the electrical activity of the heart, including the voltages generated and the time that it takes for these voltages to flow from one area of the heart to another. The ECG tracing can be used to identify the anatomical source of abnormal rhythms, the presence of inadequate blood flow (ischemia), destruction of heart muscle (infarction), enlargement of heart chambers (atrial and ventricular hypertrophy), delays in conduction of electrical current, and inflammation of the tissue surrounding the heart (pericarditis). In addition, it can be helpful in the evaluation of the effects of electrolyte disturbances, systemic diseases, and medications or drugs that act on the heart and assist in the evaluation of implanted pacemaker and defibrillator function. A normal heart cycle (see Figure 1 in Appendix) consists of a P wave, QRS complex, and T wave; a U wave also may be seen. This cycle is repeated at regular intervals. The P wave occurs with atrial depolarization, the QRS complex with ventricular depolarization, and the T wave with ventricular repolarization. The U wave represents nonspecific recovery after-potentials. The ECG is analyzed according to the following parameters: rate, rhythm, intervals, voltages, axis, and presence of abnormal waveforms.
Relevance to psychiatry and behavioral science	ECG tracings for many patients in psychiatric care show changes suggestive of ischemia, even in the absence of any clinical correlates of disease. For example, anxiety and hyperventilation may be associated with sinus tachycardia and ST-segment depression with or without T-wave inversion, possibly mediated by autonomic function. More significant ECG abnormalities are seen in patients with eating disorders with associated electrolyte derangements. In addition, a number of psychotropic medications cause ECG abnormalities. Lithium, for example, is associated with T-wave flattening or inversion in perhaps the majority of treated patients, and clozapine may be associated with ST-segment changes as well as T-wave inversion. These psychotropic-related findings are of uncertain significance. Many psychotropics are known to cause prolongation of the QT interval. Overdose of medications such as tricyclic antidepressants (TCAs) and dual-acting antidepressants may cause significant ECG changes.
Preparation of patient	The patient should abstain from smoking and avoid heavy meals for at least 30 minutes before the test, and should rest for at least 15 minutes before the test.

Electrocardiogram (ECG or EKG) *(continued)*	
Indications	• Routine admission testing for patients age 40 years and older • Preoperative screening before general anesthesia • Electroconvulsive therapy screening in patients over age 50 years or with previous abnormal ECG or known heart disease • Chest pain or other signs of possible myocardial infarction (MI) • Syncope • Irregular pulse • Initiation of a psychotropic drug that affects cardiac conduction (e.g., TCA, antipsychotic)
Reference range	*Rate*: 60–100 beats/minute *Rhythm*: Normal sinus rhythm or sinus arrhythmia *Intervals* • PR interval 120–200 milliseconds (0.12–0.20 seconds) • QRS interval 80–120 milliseconds (0.08–0.12 seconds) • QT interval 350–430 milliseconds (varies with heart rate [HR], gender, time of day) Note: Corrected QT (QTc)=QT/R-R *Voltages* • Top of R wave to bottom of S wave is 1 mV • P wave is 0.1–0.3 mV • T wave is 0.2–0.3 mV *Axis*: +90° to −30° in adult
Critical findings	*Ventricular tachycardia:* HR>100 with at least 3 irregular heartbeats in a row *Ventricular fibrillation:* very rapid HR, uncoordinated, fatal unless treated immediately *Torsades de pointes:* bradycardia, prolonged QT, and QRS that rotates around the isoelectric baseline *Severe bradycardia:* HR<40; often symptomatic

Electrocardiogram (ECG or EKG) *(continued)*	
Abnormal findings	*Bradycardia:* HR < 60
	Tachycardia: HR > 100
	Atrial fibrillation: HR is rapid, rhythm is irregular; ECG shows absence of P waves that usually precede QRS complexes.
	Atrial flutter: HR is rapid (ventricular rate about 150), QRS is narrow, ECG baseline has a "sawtooth" appearance.
	First-degree heart block: PR interval > 0.20 milliseconds; each P wave is followed by QRS.
	Second-degree heart block: Some P waves are blocked at the atrioventricular node so have no following QRS.
	Third-degree heart block (complete heart block): complete dissociation between P waves and QRS.
	QTc prolongation: > 450 milliseconds for men, > 470 milliseconds for women. Results from delayed repolarization, which enables early afterdepolarizations to occur and sets the stage for extrasystoles and possibly torsades de pointes.
	Premature ventricular contractions (PVCs) or ventricular premature depolarizations (VPDs): a wide QRS that follows closely a normal QRS. When it occurs after every normal QRS, the pattern is called bigeminy. When it occurs after every other normal QRS, the pattern is called trigeminy. When three or more PVCs occur in a row, the pattern is ventricular tachycardia.
	ST-segment changes: The normal ST segment serves as the isoelectric line on the ECG tracing. ST-segment depression (below the baseline) signifies ischemia. ST-segment elevation signifies infarction.
Interfering factors	*Age:* T-wave inversion in leads V_1–V_3 may be a normal finding into the second decade (third decade in African Americans).
	Gender: Women often exhibit slight ST-segment depression.
	Race: ST-segment elevation and T-wave inversion that disappears with maximal exercise may be seen in African Americans.
	Inaccurate lead placement affects test results.
	Reversal of limb leads may suggest infarction or dextrocardia (heart in the right chest). Deep breathing shifts the position of the heart. Variations of the normal anatomical heart position within the thorax may affect the axis. QRS axis shifts leftward with obesity, ascites, and pregnancy.
Cross-references	None

Electroencephalogram (EEG)	
Type of test	Neurophysiology
Explanation of test	The EEG records electrical potential differences between electrode pairs on the scalp or between a scalp electrode and a reference electrode. These potentials reflect underlying electrical activity in the cerebral cortex, and indirectly that of deeper structures. Electrodes are attached to the scalp in an array known as the 10-20 system, and several different patterns of electrode pairing ("montages") are captured during each EEG session. Reference electrodes are placed on the ear or mastoid, or an averaged reference is created electronically. Ideally, recordings capture the fully awake, drowsy, and sleeping states. To achieve the sleep state, the patient might require sleep deprivation on the night before the test. Several stimulation procedures are performed during the test, including hyperventilation and photic stimulation, designed to elicit epileptiform patterns. If the referring question relates to a specific provocation (e.g., seizures when listening to music), the provocation should be simulated during testing. To capture epileptiform or ictal activity arising from temporal lobes (e.g., in partial seizures), anterior temporal (T1 and T2) and ear electrodes may be used; nasopharyngeal electrodes offer no advantage and are uncomfortable for the patient. If the referring question relates to encephalopathy, the patient may require specific alerting procedures; for example, the patient may be asked to count backward from 20, or the technician might provide a tapping stimulus to maintain wakefulness for a brief interval of recording. Electroencephalographic frequencies recorded range from 0.5 Hz to approximately 35 Hz, with frequencies divided into bands as follows: delta = 0.5–4 Hz, theta = 5–8 Hz, alpha = 8–12 Hz, beta = 13–35 Hz. Higher frequencies usually represent extraneous muscle activity.
Relevance to psychiatry and behavioral science	In psychiatric practice, the EEG finds greatest utility in the diagnosis and differential diagnosis of delirium. The EEG is exquisitely sensitive to the changes in brain metabolism and activity accompanying the clinical signs and symptoms of delirium, showing generalized slow-wave activity in the delta and theta ranges, slowing of the posterior dominant frequency, disorganization of the background rhythm, and loss of reactivity to eye opening and closing. The EEG can be used to distinguish delirium from primary psychosis, as it is usually normal in the latter condition. It can be used to detect the presence of delirium superimposed on dementia, in which case the amount of slow-wave activity is greatly increased over the baseline tracing. Serial EEGs can be helpful in gauging response to treatment of delirium, with serial studies showing improvement in slowing and increase in mean frequency.

Electroencephalogram (EEG) *(continued)*

Relevance to psychiatry and behavioral science *(continued)*	Another use of the EEG in psychiatry is to aid in distinguishing seizures from pseudoseizures if the ictal event can be captured during the recording and neither spike nor spike-and-wave activity is seen. Caveats here relate to the fact that the interictal EEG may be completely normal, that patients who have pseudoseizures may also have true seizures, and that some patients who have convincing signs and symptoms but no electroencephalographic correlates may actually have deep epileptogenic foci, with activity captured only by depth recording. When the EEG is used for the workup of "mental status changes" or confusional states, it may capture nonconvulsive status epilepticus, a condition disproportionately affecting elderly women who present with an ongoing oneiric state or stupor. In these cases, the EEG shows sustained ictal activity.
	Characteristic EEG changes are also seen in sporadic Creutzfeldt-Jakob disease and in subacute sclerosing panencephalitis. The EEG may also detect toxic effects of drugs such as lithium, where a disorganized rhythm, interspersed slow-wave activity, and triphasic waves may be seen.
Preparation of patient	The patient may need reassurance that the EEG only *records* electrical activity and does not deliver an electrical stimulus. The process of electrode application should be explained; this process often includes the use of collodion, an adhesive gel that requires vigorous cleansing for removal. The patient should avoid sedatives before testing. If a hypnotic is required to capture sleep, chloral hydrate should be used in preference to other drugs. Sleep deprivation may be needed to ensure that an adequate sleep sample is obtained (e.g., in the case of suspected seizures). The sleep deprivation protocol is to awaken the patient at 4:00 A.M. and then keep the patient awake without naps or stimulants until the time of testing.
Indications	• Confirming the diagnosis of delirium • Distinguishing delirium from catatonia • Monitoring the course of delirium (serial studies) • Detecting the presence of epileptiform or ictal activity • Monitoring the efficacy of antiepileptic drugs • Diagnosing nonconvulsive status epilepticus • Incidental detection of mass lesions (neuroimaging being superior for this purpose) • Aiding in the diagnosis of Creutzfeldt-Jakob disease • Aiding in the diagnosis of subacute sclerosing panencephalitis

Electroencephalogram (EEG) *(continued)*

Indications *(continued)*	• Confirming suspected lithium toxicity • Various indications in critical care: evaluating coma, confirming brain death • Aiding in the diagnosis of somatoform presentations (e.g., suspected pseudoseizures)
Normal patterns	• Posterior dominant (alpha) frequency 8–12 Hz • Presence of beta activity during wakefulness, prominent in frontal areas • Abundant theta and delta slow-wave activity only in drowsiness and sleep • Frontal intermittent rhythmic delta activity (FIRDA) only in transitions to and from sleep • In drowsiness and light sleep: vertex sharp waves • In stage 2 sleep: sleep spindles, K complexes • No epileptiform activity or focal slowing • No abnormalities elicited by hyperventilation or photic stimulation
Abnormal patterns	Spike, spike-and-slow-wave complexes, slow waves in awake state, focal slowing, periodic patterns, triphasic waves; FIRDA outside of transitions. Abnormalities may be elicited by stimulation procedures.
Interfering factors	For electroencephalographic abnormalities that are intermittent in nature, a single EEG may prove to have low yield. This is particularly true for epileptiform or ictal (seizure) activity when the clinical manifestations do not appear during the EEG recording period or when the provoking stimulus cannot be simulated in the laboratory. For seizure activity, yield increases with sleep deprivation, greater number of electroencephalographic recordings, and longer time of recording. For this reason, it may be advised to use an ambulatory (24-hour) EEG or EEG telemetry monitoring. An electroencephalographic study that does not include wakefulness, drowsiness, and stage 2 sleep along with hyperventilation and photic stimulation is considered incomplete for detection of epileptiform activity. An electroencephalographic study that does not explicitly produce and document alerting stimuli for the patient with depressed level of consciousness (e.g., suspected delirium) is considered incomplete. Many psychotropic drugs affect the EEG, usually introducing either slow-wave activity (e.g., antipsychotics or mood stabilizers) or beta activity (e.g., sedative-hypnotics or alcohol).
Cross-reference	Delirium

Electrolytes panel	
Type of test	Blood
Explanation of test	This panel has four tests: • Sodium • Potassium • Chloride • Carbon dioxide
Relevance to psychiatry and behavioral science	This panel is used to screen and monitor for basic electrolyte abnormalities in patients treated with lithium and certain other psychotropic drugs.
Preparation of patient	None needed
Indications	• Detecting or ruling out a specific lab abnormality • Monitoring a known condition and its associated lab abnormality
Reference range	See entries for individual tests.
Critical value(s)	
Increased levels	
Decreased levels	
Interfering factors	
Cross-references	Basic Metabolic Panel (BMP) Comprehensive Metabolic Panel (CMP) See entries for individual tests.

Ethylene glycol level

Type of test	Blood
Explanation of test	Ethylene glycol is an odorless, sweet-tasting substance found in certain detergents, paints, de-icing products, brake fluid, and antifreeze. Ingestion of as little as 4 fluid ounces of ethylene glycol can kill an average-sized adult. Ethylene glycol can be accidentally ingested by children, intentionally taken in overdose, or abused as a substance in place of ethanol. The diagnosis of ethylene glycol poisoning can be made by the ethylene glycol level. The test is not available in all settings.
Relevance to psychiatry and behavioral science	Alcoholic patients without access to ethanol sometimes abuse ethylene glycol. Initial symptoms of ethylene glycol poisoning resemble those of alcohol intoxication, except that the patient's breath does not smell like alcohol.
Preparation of patient	None needed
Indications	Clinical suspicion of ethylene glycol ingestion
Reference range	The assay will not detect a level <5 mg/dL.
Critical value(s)	Toxicity is usually at levels >20 mg/dL. In susceptible individuals, any amount in plasma may be associated with toxicity.
Increased levels	• Accidental ingestion (e.g., by a child) • Intentional overdose • Abuse in place of ethanol
Decreased levels	Not applicable
Interfering factors	The plasma level may be below the assay's limit of detection even though the patient shows signs of toxicity.
Cross-references	Ethylene Glycol Poisoning Osmolality (Serum and Urine)

Barceloux DG, Krenzelok EP, Olson K, et al: American Academy of Clinical Toxicology practice guidelines on the treatment of ethylene glycol poisoning. J Toxicol Clin Toxicol 37(5):537–560, 1999

Brent J: Current management of ethylene glycol poisoning. Drugs 61(7):979–988, 2001

Flurazepam level

Type of test	Blood
Explanation of test	Benzodiazepines are Schedule IV sedative-hypnotic drugs used to treat anxiety and insomnia. Flurazepam is a rapidly acting drug with a negligible half-life for the parent compound and a very long half-life for the metabolite *N*-desalkylflurazepam. In general, metabolite levels are checked when either overdose or noncompliance is suspected or to detect use without a prescription.
Relevance to psychiatry and behavioral science	Toxicity with chronic benzodiazepine ingestion may manifest as confusion, disorientation, memory impairment, ataxia, decreased reflexes, and dysarthria. With acute overdose, the patient may exhibit somnolence, confusion, ataxia, decreased reflexes, vertigo, dysarthria, respiratory depression, and coma. More serious consequences usually involve co-ingestion of alcohol or other sedatives. If the ingestion was within 4 hours or if the patient is symptomatic, activated charcoal should be given and then repeated, because these drugs undergo hepatic recirculation. Administration of flumazenil does not affect flurazepam level.
Preparation of patient	None needed
Indications	• Screening for drug use • Suspicion of overdose • Signs of toxicity in a treated patient • Suspected noncompliance with prescribed therapy
Reference range	*N*-desalkylflurazepam: 0.01–0.24 µg/mL
Critical value(s)	*N*-desalkylflurazepam: toxic >0.30 µg/mL lethal >0.50 µg/mL
Increased levels	• Overdose • Overuse • Poor metabolism • Hepatic encephalopathy
Decreased levels	Noncompliance
Interfering factors	None
Cross-references	Benzodiazepines Drug Screen (Toxicology Screen)

Folate (also known as folic acid)	
Type of test	Blood
Explanation of test	Folate is a water-soluble vitamin with a number of important cellular and metabolic functions. Regular intake of folate is required, and it is particularly crucial during the first trimester of pregnancy to avoid neural tube defects in the developing fetus. A folate deficiency syndrome has three stages. In the first stage, the plasma folate level drops. If folate is not replaced, then the red blood cell (RBC) folate level drops. If the deficiency continues (4 months or more), then bone marrow is affected and anemia develops. This is a megaloblastic anemia, with large, immature, nonfunctioning RBCs containing excess hemoglobin.
	In the general North American population, folate deficiency is now less common because cereals, breads, and grain products are folate enriched, but the deficiency can still be seen in those with low intake of these foods as well as inadequate intake of fresh green vegetables and beans. Folate deficiency is still common in developing countries. This deficiency is also seen in specific patient populations. Malabsorption of folate (along with vitamin B_{12}) can affect individuals with disease or surgical conditions involving the small intestine, such as celiac disease or gastric bypass surgery. Accelerated loss of folate can occur in patients with liver disease, alcoholism, or kidney disease. Certain medications can decrease folate levels (including phenytoin, metformin, and methotrexate).
	RBC folate is a better indicator of folate status than is serum folate. When folate is checked, vitamin B_{12} should also be checked, because the two deficiencies can occur together.
Relevance to psychiatry and behavioral science	Low folate levels are correlated with depression and a poor response to antidepressant medication. Some patients with depression respond to folate augmentation of antidepressant medication, even when folate levels are in the normal or low-normal range. Folate levels are also correlated with dementia in certain patient populations, and folate is one of the lab tests routinely ordered in the workup of cognitive impairment. Newly admitted psychiatric patients with a variety of diagnoses are more likely than the general population to have low folate levels.
Preparation of patient	The patient should fast for 6–8 hours before the test.

Folate
(also known as folic acid) *(continued)*

Indications	• Physical symptoms that suggest folate deficiency: dizziness, weakness, fatigue, headaches, difficulty concentrating, palpitations, diarrhea, sore mouth or tongue
	• Mental or behavioral changes, especially in the elderly patient
	• Suspected malnutrition or malabsorption in patients with conditions such as alcoholism, celiac disease, Crohn's disease, or cystic fibrosis
	• Evaluation of megaloblastic anemia
Reference range	2–16 years: >160 ng/mL (>362 nmol/L)
	>16 years: 140–628 ng/mL (317–1,422 nmol/L)
Critical value(s)	None
Increased levels	• Supplementation
	• Acute renal failure
	• Active liver disease
Decreased levels	• Malabsorption: liver disease, alcoholism, gastric bypass, celiac disease
	• Use of certain medications: phenytoin, metformin, methotrexate
	• Inadequate dietary intake
	• Increased metabolism
	• Increased requirements (pregnancy)
	• Renal dialysis
	• Malignancy (lymphoproliferative disease)
	• Increased hematopoiesis (thalassemia major)
Interfering factors	RBC hemolysis, radioactive scan within 48 hours of testing, specimen handling (must be protected from light), ethnicity (values are higher in Caucasian than in African American or Mexican American individuals)
Cross-references	Alcohol Use Disorder (Alcoholism)
	Vitamin B_{12}
	Vitamin B_{12} Deficiency

Kim JM, Stewart R, Kim SW, et al: Predictive value of folate, vitamin B_{12} and homocysteine levels in late-life depression. Br J Psychiatry 192(4):268–274, 2008

Lerner V, Kanevsky M, Dwolatzky T, et al: Vitamin B_{12} and folate serum levels in newly admitted psychiatric patients. Clin Nutr 25(1):60–67, 2006

Gamma-glutamyltransferase (GGT)

Type of test	Blood
Explanation of test	The liver is the primary source of serum GGT, although the enzyme is also present in the kidney and pancreas. The enzyme is elevated in various liver diseases.
	With abstinence from drinking, GGT normalizes in 2–3 weeks. If GGT remains elevated with abstinence, further diagnostic evaluation may be warranted to exclude causes other than alcohol ingestion, such as fatty liver, biliary obstruction, cholangitis, or cholecystitis. Elevation of GGT in combination with elevation of alkaline phosphatase indicates hepatobiliary disease.
Relevance to psychiatry and behavioral science	Elevation of GGT has high sensitivity for liver disease but low specificity in the evaluation of etiology. Specificity improves through patient selection; although the GGT assay would have little use in screening for alcoholic liver disease, it would be highly useful in confirming recent drinking in a chronic drinker who is supposedly abstinent (e.g., in treatment). In men, GGT is used alone for this indication. In women, it is used in tandem with carbohydrate-deficient transferrin. Specificity also improves when elevated GGT is found in combination with an aspartate transaminase (AST) to alanine transaminase (ALT) ratio >2, which is consistent with alcoholic liver disease.
Preparation of patient	The patient should fast for 8 hours and should abstain from alcohol for 24 hours before the test.
Indications	• Detecting covert alcohol ingestion (recent drinking) • Detecting hepatobiliary disease • Monitoring progression of liver disease or liver metastases
Reference range	Adult males: 7–47 U/L (0.12–1.80 µkat/L) Adult females: 5–25 U/L (0.08–0.42 µkat/L) Elderly individuals may have slightly higher levels. Values vary with method used; consult lab reference values.
Critical value(s)	None
Increased levels	• Hepatitis • Myocardial infarction • Cirrhosis • Alcohol ingestion • Hepatic necrosis • Pancreatitis • Hepatic tumor or metastasis

Gamma-glutamyltransferase (GGT) *(continued)*	
Increased levels *(continued)*	• Diabetes, metabolic syndrome • Pancreatic cancer • Hepatotoxic drugs • Epstein-Barr virus • Cholestasis • Cytomegalovirus • Renal failure • Reye syndrome • *Drugs:* phenytoin, phenobarbital, and anticoagulants
Decreased levels	• Late pregnancy • *Drugs:* clofibrate, oral contraceptives
Interfering factors	Increased levels may be seen with excessive meat consumption.
Cross-references	Alcohol Use Disorder (Alcoholism) Alanine Transaminase (ALT) Aspartate Transaminase (AST) Carbohydrate-Deficient Transferrin (CDT or %CDT) Liver Function Tests (LFTs)

Fischbach F, Dunning MB: A Manual of Laboratory and Diagnostic Tests, 8th Edition. Philadelphia, PA, Wolters Kluwer Health/Lippincott Williams & Wilkins, 2009

Galanter M, Kleber HD, Brady KT (eds): The American Psychiatric Publishing Textbook of Substance Abuse Treatment, 5th Edition. Arlington, VA, American Psychiatric Publishing, 2015

Wu AHB: Tietz Clinical Guide to Laboratory Tests, 4th Edition. St. Louis, MO, WB Saunders, 2006

Glucose (blood sugar)	
Type of test	Blood
Explanation of test	Glucose is the body's primary source of cellular energy, obtained from carbohydrates in the diet and from conversion of glycogen stored in the liver and muscles. A constant supply of glucose is required for normal brain function. A variety of hormones regulate glucose levels, the most important of which are insulin and glucagon. Glucagon is secreted when glucose levels are low, and this results in a cascade of events that drives glucose levels up. Insulin is secreted when glucose levels are high, driving glucose into cells and lowering serum glucose levels. It is important to interpret serum levels with respect to the time of the last meal. Hyperglycemia in the fasting state suggests the diagnosis of diabetes mellitus. This can be confirmed with a glycosylated hemoglobin test or a glucose tolerance test. Hypoglycemia is most commonly seen in patients with "brittle" diabetes who have taken too much insulin. Very low blood sugar values (see panic values in the "Critical Value(s)" section below) are associated with brain damage.
Relevance to psychiatry and behavioral science	High blood glucose can be found in patients with delirium, metabolic syndrome, acute stress response, and acute pancreatitis, and in those treated with atypical antipsychotics, phenothiazines, tricyclic antidepressants (TCAs), lithium, or beta-blockers (other than propranolol). Low blood glucose can be found in patients with alcoholism, anorexia nervosa, panic attacks or other anxiety syndromes, depression, or agitation, and in patients treated with propranolol or monoamine oxidase inhibitors (MAOIs).
Preparation of patient	Optimally, the patient should fast for 8 hours before the test; water is allowed. The patient should not fast longer than 16 hours, because feedback processes may raise glucose levels. Insulin and oral hypoglycemic medications should be held until blood is drawn.
Indications	• Routine health screening • Suspicion of diabetes based on clinical signs and symptoms • Suspicion of hypoglycemia based on clinical signs and symptoms • Acute change in mental status • Workup for patients with panic attacks or unexplained anxiety • Monitoring of patients on atypical antipsychotic medications

Glucose (blood sugar) *(continued)*	
Reference range	*Fasting plasma glucose* • Adults <60 years: 74–106 mg/dL (4.1–5.9 mmol/L) • Adults 60–90 years: 82–115 mg/dL (4.6–6.4 mmol/L) • Adults >90 years: 75–121 mg/dL (4.2–6.7 mmol/L) • Children: 60–100 mg/dL (3.3–5.6 mmol/L) *Random serum glucose* • ≥1 year (of age): 70–140 mg/dL

Critical value(s)	*Diagnosis of diabetes mellitus* (World Health Organization / American Diabetes Association criteria)
	
	• Fasting ≥126 mg/dL (≥7.0 mmol/L) or
	
	• 2-hour postglucose load ≥200 mg/dL (≥11.1 mmol/L) or
	
	• Random glucose ≥200 mg/dL (≥11.1 mmol/L) plus symptoms of diabetes
	
	Panic values
	
	  Males: <50 mg/dL or >400 mg/dL
	
	  Females: <40 mg/dL or >400 mg/dL

Increased levels	• Diabetes mellitus • Acute stress response • Cushing syndrome • Pheochromocytoma • Chronic renal failure • Glucagonoma • Acute pancreatitis • Diuretic therapy • Acromegaly • Pregnancy • *Drugs:* atypical antipsychotics, TCAs, beta-blockers, corticosteroids, dextrothyroxine, diazoxide, diuretics, epinephrine, estrogens, glucagon, isoniazid, lithium, phenothiazines, phenytoin, salicylate toxicity, triamterene

Glucose (blood sugar) *(continued)*	
Decreased levels	• Insulinoma
	• Hypothyroidism
	• Hypopituitarism
	• Addison disease
	• Severe liver disease
	• Insulin overdose
	• Starvation (anorexia nervosa)
	• *Drugs:* acetaminophen, alcohol, anabolic steroids, clofibrate, disopyramide, gemfibrozil, insulin, MAOIs, pentamidine, propranolol, thiazolidinediones, sulfonylureas, biguanides, meglitinides, alpha-glucosidase inhibitors, incretin mimetics
Interfering factors	Dextrose-containing intravenous fluids
Cross-reference	Diabetes Mellitus

Hematocrit (Hct)

Type of test	Blood
Explanation of test	The hematocrit is a measure of red blood cell (RBC) mass that is either calculated from the measured hemoglobin and mean corpuscular volume or measured in a centrifuge tube and expressed as the percentage by volume of packed RBCs in whole blood. The hematocrit value is generally three times the hemoglobin value.
Relevance to psychiatry and behavioral science	A low hematocrit is associated with symptoms of fatigue, weakness, somnolence, anhedonia, and depression. A low hematocrit may be found in patients with restless legs syndrome, and symptoms of this condition may improve with interventions to raise the hematocrit. Heavy smoking and lung disease can cause secondary elevation of the hematocrit, and modification of these health risks may cause a reduction in hematocrit.
Preparation of patient	None needed
Indications	• A component of the routine complete blood count • Used to determine anemia (low hematocrit) or polycythemia (high hematocrit)
Reference range	The normal hematocrit is roughly 45%, with the following ranges: • Adult females: 36%–48% • Adult males: 42%–52%
Critical value(s)	Hct <20% associated with cardiac failure and death Hct >60% associated with spontaneous blood clotting Persistent elevation of hematocrit above the upper limit of normal for >2 months should prompt referral to hematology for evaluation. The risk of events such as large-vessel occlusion increases with hematocrit >45%.
Increased levels	• Erythrocytosis • Polycythemia vera • Shock, with hemoconcentration • Heavy smoking and lung disease

Hematocrit (Hct) *(continued)*	
Decreased levels	• Anemia
	• Leukemia, lymphoma, Hodgkin disease, myeloproliferative disorders
	• Adrenal insufficiency
	• Chronic disease
	• Acute and chronic blood loss
	• Hemolytic reaction (from incompatible blood transfusion, drug reactions, or reactions to chemicals, infections, or physical agents)
Interfering factors	Age affects hematocrit, with differing normal ranges from birth to adulthood. Patients over age 60 years tend to have lower hematocrits. Women generally have lower hematocrits than men. Pregnancy is associated with decreased hematocrit. High altitude is associated with increased hematocrit. Hematocrit values may be unreliable immediately after acute blood loss or transfusion. The hematocrit value changes linearly with change in RBC number for normal-sized cells, but when cells are microcytic or macrocytic, this relationship does not hold.
Cross-reference	Complete Blood Count (CBC)

Hemoglobin (Hb)	
Type of test	Blood
Explanation of test	Hemoglobin combines with and carries oxygen and carbon dioxide within red blood cells. The oxygen-combining capacity of the blood is directly related to the hemoglobin concentration. Hemoglobin also serves as a buffer for extracellular fluid to maintain physiological pH. The hemoglobin value is generally one-third that of the hematocrit.
Relevance to psychiatry and behavioral science	See Hematocrit (Hct) entry.
Preparation of patient	None needed
Indications	• A component of the routine complete blood count • Screening for anemia • Determining severity of anemia • Monitoring response to treatment for anemia • Evaluating polycythemia
Reference range	Children 6 months to <5 years: 11.0 g/dL (6.8 mmol/L) Children 5 to <12 years: 11.5 g/dL (7.1 mmol/L) Adolescents 12–15 years: 12.0 g/dL (7.4 mmol/L) Females >15 years: 12.0 g/dL (7.4 mmol/L) Pregnant females: 11.0 (6.8 mmol/L) Males >15 years: 13.0 (8.1 mmol/L)
Critical value(s)	<5.0 g/dL associated with heart failure and death >20 g/dL associated with capillary clogging
Increased levels	• Polycythemia vera • Congestive heart failure • Chronic obstructive pulmonary disease
Decreased levels	• Iron deficiency anemia • Thalassemia • Pernicious anemia • Hemoglobinopathies • Liver disease • Hypothyroidism • Hemorrhage

Hemoglobin (Hb) *(continued)*	
Decreased levels *(continued)*	• Hemolytic anemia (e.g., due to drug reactions, transfusion of incompatible blood, infectious disease or chemical exposure, burns, or artificial heart valves) • Systemic diseases (e.g., Hodgkin disease, leukemia, lymphoma, lupus, sarcoidosis, carcinomatosis)
Interfering factors	Increased hemoglobin is seen in those living at high altitude and with extreme exercise. Decreased hemoglobin is seen in pregnancy and with excessive fluid intake. Hemoglobin variants that may confound hemoglobin measurement include methemoglobin, sickle cell hemoglobin, fetal hemoglobin, and deoxyhemoglobin.
Cross-reference	Complete Blood Count (CBC)

Hemoglobin A$_{1C}$ (HbA$_{1C}$)

Type of test	Blood
Explanation of test	HbA$_{1C}$ is a form of glycosylated hemoglobin (hemoglobin bound to glucose) that is formed slowly over the 120-day life span of the red blood cell (RBC), with the amount formed proportional to the amount of glucose present in the blood. The HbA$_{1C}$ value reflects the average blood sugar level in the 120 days before the test, thus providing a longer-term view of blood sugar control. HbA$_{1C}$ is reported as a percentage of total hemoglobin. This test does not replace fasting blood sugar checks by blood draw or home glucose monitoring, which are required to determine whether immediate medication or dietary changes are needed. The American Diabetes Association is now recommending that HbA$_{1C}$ values be converted to estimated average glucose (eAG) values, which correspond more closely to glucose meter values. The conversion can be made using the table in the "Reference Range" section below, or by the following formula: $28.7 \times A_{1C} - 46.7 = eAG$.
Relevance to psychiatry and behavioral science	This test may be ordered routinely with admission lab tests. It may be useful in the evaluation of poor compliance with diabetic regimens, especially among adolescents. Patients with symptoms of metabolic syndrome should be considered for HbA$_{1C}$ testing.
Preparation of patient	Fasting is not necessary for the test.
Indications	Routine health maintenance in patients with diabetes (either type 1 or type 2): • Every 6 months in those meeting treatment goals, with stable glycemic control • Every 3 months in those whose treatment has been changed or who are not meeting glycemic goals
Reference range	Reference interval for nondiabetic patients: 4%–6% Target for patients with diabetes: <7% (ideal is <6.5%) Conversion of HbA$_{1C}$ to eAG values: <table><tr><td>**HbA$_{1C}$ (%)**</td><td>**eAG (mg/dL)**</td><td>**eAG (mmol/L)**</td></tr><tr><td>6</td><td>126</td><td>7.0</td></tr><tr><td>6.5</td><td>140</td><td>7.8</td></tr><tr><td>7</td><td>154</td><td>8.6</td></tr><tr><td>7.5</td><td>169</td><td>9.4</td></tr><tr><td>8</td><td>183</td><td>10.1</td></tr><tr><td>8.5</td><td>197</td><td>10.9</td></tr><tr><td>9</td><td>212</td><td>11.8</td></tr><tr><td>9.5</td><td>226</td><td>12.6</td></tr><tr><td>10</td><td>240</td><td>13.4</td></tr></table>

Hemoglobin A$_{1C}$ (HbA$_{1C}$) (continued)

Critical value(s)	8% or greater value increases the risk of diabetic complications >15% signifies that diabetes is out of control 14.3%–20% corresponds to ketoacidosis
Increased levels	• Hyperglycemia • Other conditions: iron deficiency anemia, splenectomy, alcohol toxicity, lead toxicity, polycystic ovary syndrome
Decreased levels	• Hypoglycemia (relative) • Other conditions: hemolytic anemia, chronic blood loss, pregnancy, chronic renal failure
Interfering factors	This test cannot be used to monitor diabetic control in patients with chronic renal failure because of reduced life span of RBCs. Therapeutic use of monoclonal antibodies can be associated with spuriously low levels of HbA$_{1C}$.
Cross-references	Diabetes Mellitus Glucose (Blood Sugar) Metabolic Syndrome

Saudek CD, Derr RL, Kalyani RR: Assessing glycemia in diabetes using self-monitoring blood glucose and hemoglobin A1c. JAMA 295(14):1688–1697, 2006

Steffes M, Cleary P, Goldstein D, et al: Hemoglobin A1c measurements over nearly two decades: sustaining comparable values throughout the Diabetes Control and Complications Trial and the Epidemiology of Diabetes Interventions and Complications study. Clin Chem 51:753–758, 2005

Hepatitis panel

Type of test	Blood
Explanation of test	When a patient presents with signs and symptoms suggestive of acute hepatitis but has no prior history of hepatitis, a screening panel is ordered. In the United States, screening is carried out for hepatitis A, B, and C infection simultaneously, except in the case of a known exposure to a specific type. The panel includes the following tests: • Hepatitis A virus antibody—immunoglobulin M (IgM) • Hepatitis B virus core antibody—IgM • Hepatitis B virus surface antigen with reflex to confirmation • Hepatitis C virus antibody If the patient presents with signs and symptoms suggestive of acute hepatitis and has a known history of hepatitis B infection, the patient is tested instead for co-infection with delta hepatitis (hepatitis D).
Relevance to psychiatry and behavioral science	Hepatitis is highly prevalent among patients in psychiatric care. Hepatitis B, C, and D are transmitted through body fluids. Sexual exposure is a common mode of transmission for hepatitis B but is rare for hepatitis C. Needle sharing is the most common mode of transmission for hepatitis C, but hepatitis B also can be transmitted in this way. Hepatitis A is generally a mild, self-limited disease, whereas hepatitis B, C, and D may cause acute liver failure or become chronic and lead to cirrhosis or hepatocellular carcinoma.
Preparation of patient	None needed
Indications	• New-onset jaundice, dark urine, nausea, and/or anorexia • Exposure to hepatitis • Elevated liver enzymes • Suspicion of chronic hepatitis
Reference range	Negative testing for hepatitis A antibody (Ab), hepatitis B core Ab and surface antigen (Ag), and hepatitis C Ab
Critical value(s)	None

Hepatitis panel *(continued)*	
Positive test	• Hepatitis A Ab positive: acute hepatitis A
	• Hepatitis B Ab positive and surface Ag positive: acute hepatitis B or chronic hepatitis (Consider hepatitis B virus DNA testing.)
	• Hepatitis C Ab positive: acute hepatitis C or chronic hepatitis (For high positive, do RNA quantitative testing; for low positive, do recombinant immunoblot assay.)
Negative test	See "Reference Range" section above.
Interfering factors	Hemolyzed or lipemic specimens, those containing particulate material, or heat-inactivated specimens invalidate results.
Cross-reference	Hepatitis (Viral)

Bart G, Piccolo P, Zhang L, et al: Markers for hepatitis A, B and C in methadone maintained patients: an unexpectedly high co-infection with silent hepatitis B. Addiction 103(4):681–686, 2008

National Institutes of Health Consensus Statement on Management of Hepatitis C: 2002. NIH Consens State Sci Statements 19:1–46, 2002

HIV testing

Type of test	Blood
Explanation of test	Most HIV infections in the United States are HIV-1; HIV-2 is endemic to West Africa. With infection, the virus localizes to lymphoid tissues, infecting CD4$^+$ helper cells and T-cell lymphocytes. Office-based rapid screening tests may be used initially (e.g., the Clearview HIV 1/2 STAT-PAK, the Med-Mira Reveal Rapid HIV-1 Antibody Test, or the Uni-Gold Recombigen HIV). These tests are more than 99% sensitive and specific, and results become positive 3–5 weeks after infection. Alternatively, laboratory-based screening consists of HIV-1/2 combined antibodies with reflex to HIV-1 confirmation by Western blot. These tests also become positive 3–5 weeks after infection. Treatment for HIV is monitored using quantitative viral load, CD4$^+$ count, and drug resistance testing (genotyping). Treatment is initiated for patients with CD4$^+$ count <350 and/or RNA (viral load) >100,000 and is considered for other patients.
Relevance to psychiatry and behavioral science	The Centers for Disease Control and Prevention recommends HIV screening for all patients ages 13–64, annual screening for high-risk patients, and routine prenatal screening. High-risk patients include intravenous drug users, those with multiple sexual encounters, and those with tuberculosis, chronic hepatitis, or recurrent pneumonia.
Preparation of patient	Patient counseling is mandatory with HIV testing. The following information should be provided to the patient, whether for an office-based or a laboratory-based test: information about the HIV test, its benefits and consequences, ways HIV is transmitted and how it can be prevented, the meaning of the test results, and where to obtain further information and other services, including treatment. Those tested with rapid tests should be informed that results will be available during the visit and that confirmatory testing will be needed if the rapid test is positive. In this case, a return visit should be scheduled to discuss the confirmatory test results.
Indications	See "Relevance to Psychiatry and Behavioral Science" section above.
Negative test	Not HIV
Positive test	Testing is repeated to confirm HIV.
Indeterminate test	This result is usually caused by cross-reacting antibodies in an uninfected patient. The patient should be retested in 4–8 weeks, and then again in 6 months.

HIV testing *(continued)*	
Interfering factors	If the patient is tested too soon after exposure, the test may be negative. Cross-reacting antibodies may cause a false-positive result.
Cross-reference	HIV/AIDS

Price RW, Epstein LG, Becker JT, et al: Biomarkers of HIV-1 CNS infection and injury. Neurology 69(18):1781–1788, 2007

Syed Iqbal H, Balakrishnan P, Murugavel KG, et al: Performance characteristics of a new rapid immunochromatographic test for the detection of antibodies to human immunodeficiency virus (HIV) types 1 and 2. J Clin Lab Anal 22(3):178–185, 2008

Lipase	
Type of test	Blood
Explanation of test	Lipase is an enzyme released by the pancreas into the small intestine that is involved in the metabolism of fats to free fatty acids and glycerol. With pancreatic injury, lipase appears in the circulation shortly after amylase and remains elevated for a longer period (a week or more). An elevated lipase level is more specific to pancreatic disease than is an elevated amylase level. The lipase level is normal in patients with elevated amylase who have peptic ulcer disease, salivary adenitis, inflammatory bowel disease, intestinal obstruction, or macroamylasemia.
Relevance to psychiatry and behavioral science	Lipase is elevated along with amylase in pancreatitis, and certain populations are at particular risk for this condition, including patients with alcoholism (especially males), gallstones (especially females), and hyperlipidemia, and those treated with medications such as valproate, corticosteroids, or isoniazid (INH). Elevated lipase can help in evaluating the cause of elevated amylase, which can be increased from salivary sources (e.g., eating disorders with purging) and in other conditions noted above.
Preparation of patient	None needed
Indications	• Clinical suspicion of pancreatitis: epigastric or abdominal pain/tenderness with nausea and vomiting • Used with amylase to diagnose and monitor treatment of acute pancreatitis and to distinguish pancreatitis from other abdominal disorders
Reference range	Normal values vary according to testing method; consult lab report. Adults ≤60 years: 10–140 U/L (0.17–2.3 μkat/L) Adults >60 years: 18–180 U/L (0.30–3.0 μkat/L)
Critical value(s)	>600 IU/L (>10 μkat/L)
Increased levels	• Pancreatitis (alcoholic or nonalcoholic) • Pancreatic carcinoma • Cholecystitis • Hemodialysis • Bowel infarction • Peritonitis • Primary biliary cirrhosis • Chronic renal failure

Lipase *(continued)*	
Increased levels *(continued)*	• *Drugs:* clozapine, desipramine, donepezil, mirtazapine, risperidone, valproate, many opioids, and numerous nonpsychotropics, including acetaminophen, nonsteroidal anti-inflammatory drugs, isoniazid (INH), and steroids
Decreased levels	• *Drugs:* calcium, hydroxyurea, mesalamine, protamine, and somatostatin
Interfering factors	EDTA (ethylenediaminetetraacetic acid) anticoagulant used in specimen collection can interfere with test result.
Cross-reference	Amylase

Lipid panel	
Type of test	Blood
Explanation of test	The lipid panel includes total cholesterol, low-density lipoprotein cholesterol (LDL-C), high-density lipoprotein cholesterol (HDL-C), and triglycerides. In the standard panel, LDL-C is calculated from the total cholesterol, HDL-C, and triglyceride content using the Friedewald equation. This estimate of LDL-C is only accurate if the triglyceride content is less than 400 mg/dL. If the triglyceride content exceeds this limit, the extended panel is recommended, in which LDL-C is measured directly. For a number of years, LDL-C has been the primary target for intervention. Guidelines published in 2013 by the American College of Cardiology and the American Heart Association called this into question because of a lack of randomized trials that specifically evaluated treatment targets. The issue has been controversial, and more recent publications have refocused attention on LDL-C and variables such as percent reduction in LDL-C. The most recent European guidelines (2016) are in line with LDL-C reference ranges noted below. ALDL-C and coronary heart disease risk are highly correlated over a broad range of LDL levels, from low to high. If the testing is nonfasting, only the total cholesterol and HDL-C will be usable. In this case, if the cholesterol is ≥200 mg/dL or the HDL-C is <40 mg/dL, then a follow-up fasting profile is required to determine LDL-C. HDL-C level is inversely related to coronary risk; intervention may be indicated when this value is low. The very low density lipoprotein level (VLDL) can be estimated by dividing the triglyceride value (mg/dL) by 5. This calculation is invalidated by high triglyceride levels (>400 mg/dL). As with triglycerides, increased levels of VLDL have been found to correlate with increased risk of heart disease and stroke.
Relevance to psychiatry and behavioral science	Many psychotropic medications—particularly atypical anti-psychotics and antidepressants—have adverse effects on cholesterol levels. In addition, certain psychiatric patient populations are at high risk of lipid abnormalities, obesity, and the metabolic syndrome. For these reasons, it is imperative that psychiatrists and other mental health professionals become knowledgeable about lipid measurement as well as target lipid levels and interventions needed to achieve them. In current practice, the primary therapeutic target is LDL-C. Lifestyle interventions that lower LDL-C include the following: • Brisk aerobic exercise 30 minutes/day most days of the week • Smoking cessation

Lipid panel *(continued)*	
Relevance to psychiatry and behavioral science *(continued)*	• Weight loss if overweight/obese • No more than moderate alcohol intake • Diet rich in n-3 polyunsaturated fatty acids (oils, nuts, cold-water fish, shellfish), with limited high-glycemic-index carbohydrates
Preparation of patient	The patient should fast for 9–12 hours before the test. An initial nonfasting test may be acceptable, but if the values are abnormal, a follow-up fasting test will be needed. The patient should abstain from alcohol for 24 hours before the test. A diet containing consistent levels of cholesterol should be consumed for 3 weeks before the test. Drugs that affect cholesterol levels (e.g., statins) should be withheld for 24 hours before the test.
Indications	• Routine health screening for all adults 20 years of age, obtained every 5 years • Lipid profile 1–3 months after intervention (lipid-lowering drug or lifestyle modification) • Lipid profile annually in patients on lipid-lowering drugs with optimal effect • Lipid profile annually in patients with diabetes

Reference range	*Adults*
	
	    Total cholesterol <200 mg/dL
	
	    LDL cholesterol <100 mg/dL (<70 mg/dL with history of cardiovascular event)
	
	    HDL cholesterol ≥40 mg/dL
	
	    Triglycerides <150 mg/dL
	
	Children and adolescents
	
	    Total cholesterol ≤169 mg/dL
	
	    LDL cholesterol ≤109 mg/dL

Critical value(s)	*Adults*
	
	    Total cholesterol ≥240 mg/dL
	
	    LDL cholesterol ≥160 mg/dL
	
	    HDL cholesterol ≤39 mg/dL
	
	    Triglycerides ≥200 mg/dL
	
	Children and adolescents
	
	    Total cholesterol ≥200 mg/dL
	
	    LDL cholesterol ≥130 mg/dL

Lipid panel *(continued)*	
Increased levels	• Familial hyperlipidemia • Glycogen storage disease • Coronary heart disease • Obstructive liver disease • Primary biliary cirrhosis • Nephrotic syndrome • Chronic renal failure • Cushing syndrome • Diabetes, type 2 • Anorexia nervosa • Hypothyroidism • Obesity • Pregnancy • *Drugs:* carbamazepine, steroids, levodopa, phenothiazines, HIV protease inhibitors, and phenytoin
Decreased levels	• Tangier disease • Abetalipoproteinemia, hypobetalipoproteinemia • Hepatocellular necrosis • Hepatitis • Porphyria • Tuberculosis • Malignancy • Hyperthyroidism • Malabsorption • Malnutrition • Severe acute illness • Cirrhosis • Depression, suicidal behavior • Epilepsy • Pernicious anemia • Inflammation • Infection • *Drugs:* haloperidol, monoamine oxidase inhibitors, and thyroid hormone

Lipid panel *(continued)*	
Interfering factors	High triglyceride concentrations affect the accuracy of methods used by many laboratories to calculate LDL-C.
Cross-references	Metabolic Syndrome
	Triglycerides

Bangalore S, Fayyad R, Kastelein JJ, et al: 2013 Cholesterol guidelines revisited: percent LDL cholesterol reduction or attained LDL cholesterol level or both for prognosis? Am J Med 129:384–391, 2016

National Cholesterol Education Program (NCEP) Expert Panel on Detection, Evaluation, and Treatment of High Blood Cholesterol in Adults (Adult Treatment Panel III): Third Report of the National Cholesterol Education Program (NCEP) Expert Panel on Detection, Evaluation, and Treatment of High Blood Cholesterol in Adults (Adult Treatment Panel III) final report. Circulation 106(25):3143–3421, 2002

National Guideline Clearinghouse (NGC): Guideline summary: 2013 ACC/AHA guideline on the treatment of blood cholesterol to reduce atherosclerotic cardiovascular risk in adults: a report of the American College of Cardiology/American Heart Association Task Force on Practice Guidelines. Rockville, MD, National Guideline Clearinghouse, Agency for Healthcare Research and Quality, July 1, 2014. Available at: https://www.guideline.gov/summaries/summary/48337/2013-accaha-guideline-on-the-treatment-of-blood-cholesterol-to-reduce-atherosclerotic-cardiovascular-risk-in-adults-a-report-of-the-american-college-of-cardiologyamerican-heart-association-task-force-on-practice-guidelines. Accessed August 29, 2016.

Piepoli MF, Hoes AW, Agewall S, et al: 2016 European guidelines on cardiovascular disease prevention in clinical practice: The Sixth Joint Task Force of the European Society of Cardiology and Other Societies on Cardiovascular Disease Prevention in Clinical Practice. Eur Heart J 37:2315–2381, 2016

Lithium level	
Type of test	Blood
Explanation of test	Lithium is an alkali metal salt used to treat bipolar disorder and mood instability in the context of dementia and other neuropsychiatric conditions. When the lithium level is checked, blood should be drawn 12 hours after the last dose (trough) for proper interpretation of results.
Relevance to psychiatry and behavioral science	Lithium toxicity can be acute, chronic, or acute-on-chronic. With acute toxicity, gastrointestinal symptoms are prominent, the correlation of lithium level with signs and symptoms is poor, and rapid recovery on holding the drug is the rule. With chronic toxicity, central nervous system symptoms are more prominent, and renal, cardiac, and thyroid effects are seen. Also with chronic toxicity, the correlation of lithium level with signs and symptoms is relatively good. With mild toxicity (level ~1.5 mEq/L), nausea, vomiting, diarrhea, and coarsening of tremor may be seen. As toxicity worsens (~2.0 mEq/L), dysarthria and hyperreflexia may be noted. At higher levels (~2.5 mEq/L), abnormal movements such as myoclonus, ataxia, and confusion may be seen. When the lithium level is >3.0 mEq/L, seizures, delirium, and coma may develop. Dialysis should be considered for patients with very high serum levels or rising serum levels and for those with renal failure who are unable to excrete lithium.
Preparation of patient	The patient should be instructed to hold lithium until after blood is drawn, and the phlebotomy appointment should be scheduled as closely as possible to the 12-hour mark described in the "Explanation of Test" section above.
Indications	• Signs/symptoms of lithium toxicity • Routine monitoring of lithium therapy • When lithium is started or a change is made in the dose, levels should be checked within 1 week, and then every 2–3 months for the first 6 months of treatment. After 6 months, levels should be checked every 6–12 months. Other lab tests needed for screening and monitoring of lithium therapy are noted in Lithium entry in Chapter 3, "Psychotropic Medications."
Reference range	Adult: 0.5–1.2 mmol/L (1 mmol=1 mEq) Geriatric: 0.4–1.0 mmol/L
Critical value(s)	≥1.6 mmol/L

Lithium level *(continued)*	
Increased levels	<ul><li>Overdose</li><li>Acute renal insufficiency or failure</li><li>Sodium restriction</li><li>Coadministration of angiotensin-converting enzyme (ACE) inhibitors, thiazide diuretics, nonsteroidal anti-inflammatory drugs, or fluoxetine</li></ul>
Decreased levels	Coadministration of sodium chloride, sodium bicarbonate, psyllium, fleawort or fleabane (herbals), acetazolamide, aminophylline, or theophylline
Interfering factors	Collection of blood into a lithium-heparin tube will cause a spurious elevation in level.
Cross-reference	Manic Episode

Liver function tests (LFTs)	
Type of test	Blood
Explanation of test	The panel used to screen for liver dysfunction usually includes alanine transaminase (ALT), aspartate transaminase (AST), alkaline phosphatase (ALP), direct and total serum bilirubin, albumin, and prothrombin time (PT). The tests can be grouped conceptually as follows: • Tests of hepatocellular injury—ALT and AST • Tests of cholestasis—ALP • Tests of excretory function—bilirubin (direct and total) • Tests of biosynthetic function—albumin and PT The first two categories do not measure liver function, but instead indicate the type of liver disease: hepatocellular versus cholestatic. The use of a panel of tests increases both sensitivity and specificity. When all tests are normal, the probability of liver disease is low. When more than one test is abnormal, or when abnormalities persist on serial testing, the probability increases. The inclusion of biosynthetic tests helps minimize false-negative test results in patients with advanced hepatocellular injury (e.g., alcoholic cirrhosis), in whom AST and ALT values may be normal or low. It should be noted, however, that albumin can be low and PT prolonged for reasons other than liver disease. Tests used to follow up on screening abnormalities include gamma-glutamyltransferase (GGT), to aid in determining whether ALP elevations are due to liver disease; hepatitis serology, to determine type of viral hepatitis; and autoimmune markers.
Relevance to psychiatry and behavioral science	LFTs may be abnormal in a number of conditions encountered in psychiatry, including alcoholism, hepatitis B and C viral infections, metabolic syndrome, and Wilson disease. Drugs of abuse that may cause abnormal LFTs include cocaine, 3,4-methylenedioxymethamphetamine (MDMA; Ecstasy), phencyclidine (PCP), toluene inhalants, and anabolic steroids. Many herbal and alternative medical remedies affect the liver, and these substances are often overlooked as potential culprits. Especially problematic from a liver function standpoint are the herbs chaparral, gentian, skullcap, germander, alchemilla, and senna. A variety of Chinese herbs are implicated as well, as is shark cartilage. Numerous prescribed medications are known to affect LFTs, including all classes of psychotropic drugs.

Liver function tests (LFTs) *(continued)*

Relevance to psychiatry and behavioral science *(continued)*	AST and ALT often increase early in the course of treatment with a psychotropic drug or with a dose increase. This is not necessarily an indication for drug discontinuation. If AST and ALT values are less than three times the baseline and ALP and bilirubin are normal, LFTs can simply be checked weekly. When values plateau, testing intervals can be lengthened. If AST and/or ALT values rise to more than three times the baseline or more than two times the upper limit of normal, the drug should be stopped and/or gastroenterology consultation obtained. Other indications for drug discontinuation include elevation of ALP or bilirubin, PT prolongation, and clinical signs/symptoms of hepatotoxicity.
Preparation of patient	None needed
Indications	• Routine health screening (with comprehensive metabolic panel) • Signs/symptoms of liver dysfunction, including jaundice, change in urine or stool color, nausea, vomiting, and/or diarrhea, hematemesis, loss of appetite, change in weight, right upper quadrant pain, ascites, abnormal bleeding, or unexplained fatigue • History of alcohol overuse • Exposure to hepatitis • Exposure to hepatotoxic drug(s) or chemicals • Monitoring liver dysfunction
Reference range	See entries for individual LFTs.
Critical value(s)	See entries for individual LFTs.
Abnormal test	In asymptomatic patients, the most common causes of abnormal LFTs are fatty liver, alcohol-related liver injury, and chronic viral hepatitis. If the pattern is one of hepatocellular injury, follow-up includes the following: • Review of drug list • Hepatitis screening • Iron, total iron-binding capacity, ferritin • Antinuclear antibody testing, serum protein electrophoresis • Ceruloplasmin (for patients <40 years)

Liver function tests (LFTs) *(continued)*	
Abnormal test *(continued)*	If the pattern is one of cholestasis, follow-up includes the following: • Review of drug list • Ultrasound of biliary system
Interfering factors	See entries for individual LFTs.
Cross-references	Alanine Transaminase (ALT) Albumin Alcohol Use Disorder (Alcoholism) Alkaline Phosphatase (ALP) Aspartate Transaminase (AST) Bilirubin Hepatitis (Viral) Metabolic Syndrome

Gopal DV, Rosen HR: Abnormal findings on liver function tests: interpreting results to narrow the diagnosis and establish a prognosis. Postgrad Med 107:100–102, 105–109, 113–114, 2000

Johnston DE: Special considerations in interpreting liver function tests. Am Fam Physician 59(8):2223–2230, 1999

Theal RM, Scott K: Evaluating asymptomatic patients with abnormal liver function test results. Am Fam Physician 53(6):2111–2119, 1996

Lorazepam level

Type of test	Blood
Explanation of test	Benzodiazepines are Schedule IV sedative-hypnotic drugs used to treat anxiety and insomnia. Lorazepam is an intermediate-acting drug with a half-life of less than a day, with no active metabolites. It is not extensively metabolized in the liver. In general, levels are checked when either overdose or noncompliance is suspected or to detect use without a prescription.
Relevance to psychiatry and behavioral science	Lorazepam is often a drug of choice among sedatives for a variety of psychiatric indications. Toxicity with chronic benzodiazepine ingestion may manifest as confusion, disorientation, memory impairment, ataxia, decreased reflexes, and dysarthria. With acute overdose, the patient may exhibit somnolence, confusion, ataxia, decreased reflexes, vertigo, dysarthria, respiratory depression, and coma. More serious consequences usually involve co-ingestion of alcohol or other sedatives. If the ingestion was within 4 hours or if the patient is symptomatic, activated charcoal should be given and then repeated, because these drugs undergo hepatic recirculation. Administration of flumazenil does not affect drug level.
Preparation of patient	None needed
Indications	• Screening for drug use • Suspicion of overdose • Signs of toxicity in a treated patient • Suspected noncompliance with prescribed therapy
Reference range	50–240 ng/mL (with dosage up to 10 mg daily)
Critical value(s)	Toxicity >300 ng/mL
Increased levels	• Overdose • Overuse
Decreased levels	Noncompliance
Interfering factors	None
Cross-reference	Drug Screen (Toxicology Screen)

Magnesium (Mg⁺⁺)

Type of test	Blood
Explanation of test	Magnesium is required for protein synthesis, carbohydrate metabolism, nucleic acid synthesis, cellular transport (e.g., of calcium, sodium, and potassium), and neuromuscular function. Magnesium combines with calcium and phosphorus to form bone. Along with other ions, it helps regulate clotting. Magnesium and calcium are closely linked in function and are tightly co-regulated. Magnesium is required for calcium to be absorbed by the intestine and also has a role in calcium metabolism. With magnesium deficiency, calcium is removed from bone and can cause calcification of the aorta and kidney. Under normal conditions, only about 1% of total body magnesium is present in serum. Decreased renal function can be associated with increased serum levels. Magnesium comes from the diet, with levels in the body regulated by control of absorption from the gastrointestinal tract and excretion through the kidneys. Abnormal levels may be seen when either of these controls is compromised. When magnesium levels are low, potassium levels are often also low. Calcium regulation is also affected by low magnesium levels, such that a low calcium level may be difficult to correct when magnesium is low.
Relevance to psychiatry and behavioral science	Alcoholism and anorexia nervosa can be associated with very low magnesium levels, which may manifest as agitation, delirium, or seizures. Lithium use, abuse of laxatives, and overuse of antacids can be associated with high magnesium levels, which may manifest as a delirium of subacute onset.
Preparation of patient	The patient should fast for 4 hours before the test.
Indications	<ul><li>A component of the admission lab workup, to evaluate electrolyte status</li><li>Symptoms of an abnormally low magnesium level such as muscle weakness, twitching, cramping, confusion, cardiac arrhythmia, or seizures</li><li>Workup for malnutrition, diarrhea, or suspected malabsorption</li><li>Evaluating acute illness in a patient with alcoholism</li><li>Monitoring renal function</li><li>Monitoring the effects of intravenous replacement of magnesium</li><li>Monitoring the effects of calcium supplementation (along with calcium and phosphorus)</li><li>Workup of chronically low levels of calcium and potassium</li></ul>

Magnesium (Mg⁺⁺) *(continued)*

Reference range	*Fasting serum levels* 　Adults <60 years: 1.6–2.6 mg/dL (0.66–1.07 mmol/L) 　Adults 60–90 years: 1.6–2.4 mg/dL (0.66–0.99 mmol/L) 　Adults >90 years: 1.7–2.3 mg/dL (0.70–0.95 mmol/L) 　Children: 1.7–2.1 mg/dL (0.70–0.86 mmol/L)
Critical value(s)	Hypomagnesemia <1.2 mg/dL (<0.49 mmol/L): tetany Hypermagnesemia >5.0 mg/dL (>2.1 mmol/L) Symptoms progress as level increases: • 5–10 mg/dL: central nervous system depression, nausea, vomiting • 10–15 mg/dL: coma, electrocardiographic changes, respiratory paralysis • 30 mg/dL: complete heart block • 34–40 mg/dL: cardiac arrest
Increased levels	• Oversupplementation or overuse of magnesium-containing medications, including antacids and laxatives • Prolonged lithium or salicylate therapy • Renal failure or insufficiency (acute or chronic) • Low urine output • Dehydration • Hypothyroidism • Addison disease or adrenalectomy • Severe diabetic ketoacidosis
Decreased levels	• Low dietary intake (in the elderly, those who are malnourished, or those with alcoholism) • Malabsorption due to gastrointestinal disorders (e.g., Crohn's disease) • Excessive body fluid loss (e.g., diuretic abuse, diarrhea) • Alcoholism with cirrhosis • Chronic renal disease • Preeclampsia • Uncontrolled diabetes, diabetic ketoacidosis • Hemodialysis • Tissue trauma (surgery or burns)

Magnesium (Mg⁺⁺) *(continued)*

Interfering factors	Hemolysis invalidates results. Upright posture increases level by 4%. Calcium gluconate and other drugs can falsely decrease levels. Levels are normally low in pregnancy after the first trimester.
Cross-references	Alcohol Use Disorder (Alcoholism)
	Anorexia Nervosa
	Eating Disorders

Dørup I: Magnesium and potassium deficiency. Its diagnosis, occurrence and treatment in diuretic therapy and its consequences for growth, protein synthesis and growth factors. Acta Physiol Scand Suppl 618:1–55, 1994

Dyckner T, Wester PO: Magnesium deficiency: guidelines for diagnosis and substitution therapy. Acta Med Scand Suppl 661:37–41, 1982

Magnetic resonance imaging (MRI)	
Type of test	Imaging
Explanation of test	MRI uses a superconducting magnet and radiofrequency signals to form detailed images of the brain and other central nervous system structures. The patient is positioned supine on a flat table for the procedure, which takes approximately 45 minutes. In the closed MRI, the patient's head and upper body are inside a narrow tube, and this can cause problems for claustrophobic patients. In the open MRI, the sides of the gantry do not obstruct the patient's view, so the patient feels less confined. The open MRI is also more suitable for obese patients. The problem with open MRI is low magnet strengths; magnets used in clinical settings range from 1.5 to 3.0 T for closed systems and 0.2 to 0.35 T for open systems. In general, the stronger the magnet, the better the image resolution. Research studies are now done with extremely strong magnets of 7.0 T or more. Throughout the MRI procedure, a loud tapping noise is heard that may be mitigated somewhat by headphones. The study usually includes a sagittal T1-weighted image, axial T1-, T2-, and diffusion-weighted images, and fluid-attenuated inversion recovery (FLAIR) images throughout the brain without contrast; and coronal T1-weighted SPGR (spoiled gradient recalled) and axial T1-weighted spin echo images with contrast. The contrast agent used is gadolinium, which is administered intravenously to enhance visualization of lesions such as stroke, tumor, and abscess. Diffusion-weighted MRI is of particular value in acute stroke, because it delineates areas of early ischemia that will progress to infarction in the absence of intervention. In general, T1-weighted images are used to identify anatomy, and T2-weighted images are used to identify white matter disease. Brain MRI is superior to head computed tomography (CT) in the detection of ischemia and demyelination. It is also better for viewing brain stem and posterior fossa structures. MRI is preferred to CT in identifying lesions representing seizure focus, nonmeningeal tumors, and vascular malformations. MRI is about twice as expensive as CT, and it is not universally available for clinical use during the nighttime hours.

Magnetic resonance imaging (MRI) *(continued)*

Relevance to psychiatry and behavioral science	Characteristic MRI findings in schizophrenia include reduced total cerebral volume and atrophy of temporal lobe(s); subcortical and limbic structures may or may not show abnormalities. Characteristic MRI findings in affective disorders include areas of high signal intensity in white matter, volume loss in prefrontal cortex, and alterations in subcortical and limbic structures. In attention-deficit/hyperactivity disorder (ADHD), a 3%–4% reduction in total cerebral and cerebellar volumes, thinning of the medial prefrontal cortex, and volume reduction in dorsal anterior cingulate cortex are characteristic. In unmedicated children with ADHD, decreased white matter volume is seen.
Preparation of patient	No pretest preparation is needed. MRI will not be performed on patients with implanted metal devices, including pacemakers, defibrillators, cochlear implants, metal heart valves, pumps, neurostimulators, certain prostheses, and certain intrauterine devices. For surgical implants that are MRI compatible, the brand, style, and serial number will be requested to confirm compatibility. MRI is not advised for pregnant patients or patients with epilepsy.
Indications	• Dementia evaluation (without or with and without contrast) • Suspected normal-pressure hydrocephalus (without or with and without contrast) • Suspected Huntington's disease (without contrast) • Suspected neurodegenerative disease with brain iron accumulation (without contrast) • Parkinsonian syndrome with atypical features (without contrast) • Motor neuron disease (brain and spine without contrast) • Suspected carotid or vertebral dissection (with and without contrast, with diffusion-weighted sequences) • Ipsilateral Horner syndrome (with and without contrast, with diffusion-weighted sequences) • Sudden-onset unilateral headache (with and without contrast, with diffusion-weighted sequences) • New headache in patient over age 60 years with suspected temporal arteritis (without contrast) • New headache in HIV-positive patient (with or without contrast) • New headache in pregnant patient (without contrast)

Magnetic resonance imaging (MRI) *(continued)*	
Indications *(continued)*	• New headache with suspected meningitis/encephalitis (with and without contrast) • Transient ischemic attack involving carotid or vertebrobasilar territories (combined with magnetic resonance angiography [MRA]) • New focal neurological deficit (combined with MRA) • Parenchymal hemorrhage • Ataxia, slowly progressive (with and without contrast) • Ataxia, acute (with or without contrast; with MRA)
Normal result	• Normal structures (pituitary gland and corpus callosum) • No herniation of cerebellar tonsils • No evidence of mass lesions, hemorrhage, or acute ischemic injury • No abnormality of gray or white matter on FLAIR images • No abnormal fluid collections or displacement of midline structures • No areas of abnormal enhancement with contrast • Normal flow voids in major arteries • Normal visualized portions of the paranasal sinus, orbits, and mastoids • No abnormality of the calvarium
Abnormal result	• Periventricular or subcortical white matter changes (indicating ischemia) • Stroke, acute or old • Hemorrhage • Focal or regional atrophy • Generalized atrophy (moderate to severe) • Ventricular dilatation (hydrocephalus) • Vascular abnormalities (aneurysms, arteriovenous malformations) • Vasculitis • Neoplasm, abscess, or other mass lesion • Findings of specific infectious diseases: toxoplasmosis, tuberculosis, or herpes encephalitis

Magnetic resonance imaging (MRI) *(continued)*	
Interfering factors	Perivascular spaces (Virchow-Robin spaces) can be mistaken for lacunar infarcts. These spaces are filled with interstitial fluid and are isointense with ventricles. Virchow-Robin spaces appear as round, oval, or linear (depending on the plane of section), usually 5 mm or less, although they can be larger. *Usually, Virchow-Robin spaces are suppressed completely on FLAIR images.*
Cross-reference	Cranial Computed Tomography (Head CT or CAT Scan)

Agarwal N, Port JD, Bazzocchi M, et al: Update on the use of MR for assessment and diagnosis of psychiatric diseases. Radiology 255(1):23–41, 2010

National Guideline Clearinghouse: ACR Appropriateness Criteria. Available at: http://www.ngc .gov. Accessed May 2010.

Mean corpuscular volume (MCV)

Type of test	Blood
Explanation of test	The MCV is the volume occupied by a single red blood cell (RBC), expressed in cubic micrometers (1 μm^3=1 fL). The cell size can be normal (normocytic), smaller than normal (microcytic), or larger than normal (macrocytic). The MCV can be measured directly by an automated cell counter or computed from the hematocrit (Hct) and RBC count: $$MCV=Hct\,(\%) \times 10/RBC \text{ count } (\times 10^{12}/L)$$ One of the important uses of the MCV is to aid the differential diagnosis of macrocytic anemia, of which there are two types: megaloblastic anemia (with hypersegmented neutrophils and macrocytes in the blood or megaloblasts in the marrow) and nonmegaloblastic anemia, in which DNA synthesis is not altered and the elevation of the MCV tends to be milder, in the range of 100–110 fL.
Relevance to psychiatry and behavioral science	A number of conditions relevant to clinical psychiatry are associated with an elevation in the MCV. These include alcoholism, liver disease/cirrhosis, vitamin B_{12} or folate deficiency, smoking, and hypothyroidism. The greater the MCV elevation, the more likely that it is due to vitamin B_{12} and/or folate deficiency.
Preparation of patient	None needed
Indications	A component of the complete blood count (red cell index)
Reference range	*Adults 18–44 years* Males: 80–99 fL Females: 81–100 fL *Adults 45–64 years* Males: 81–101 fL Females: 81–101 fL *Adults 65–74 years* Males: 81–103 fL Females: 81–102 fL
Critical value(s)	None
Increased levels	• Excessive alcohol intake • Megaloblastic anemia (e.g., vitamin B_{12} or folate deficiency) • Nonmegaloblastic anemia (e.g., acute blood loss, hemolysis, liver disease, disseminated malignancy)

Mean corpuscular volume (MCV) *(continued)*	
Increased levels *(continued)*	• Smoking • Advanced age • Postmenopause • *Drugs:* anticonvulsants, aspirin, acyclovir, isoniazid (INH), metformin, chemotherapeutic agents, neomycin, colchicine, triamterene, nitrofurantoin, oral contraceptives, trimethoprim, and zidovudine, among others
Decreased levels	• Hypochromic, microcytic anemia (e.g., iron deficiency, anemia of chronic disease, thalassemia) • Certain hemoglobinopathies • Hypothyroidism (occasional)
Interfering factors	The MCV value is not reliable in the presence of a large number of reticulocytes, abnormal erythrocytes (e.g., sickle cells), a dimorphic population of erythrocytes, cold agglutinins, or a marked leukocytosis.
Cross-references	Alcohol Use Disorder (Alcoholism) Complete Blood Count (CBC) Folate Deficiency Vitamin B_{12} Deficiency

Methanol level

Type of test	Blood
Explanation of test	Methanol, known by the popular name of *wood alcohol*, is an extremely toxic substance found in antifreeze, shellac, varnish, paint thinner, fuel additives, de-icing fluids, and copy machine fluids. It may be ingested accidentally, taken in overdose intentionally, or abused by alcoholics without access to ethanol. As little as 2 tablespoons can be lethal for a child, and 2 fluid ounces for an adult. The prognosis with poisoning depends on the amount ingested and how soon treatment is administered.
Relevance to psychiatry and behavioral science	Alcoholic patients without access to ethanol sometimes abuse methanol. Like ethanol, methanol is a central nervous system depressant. The first symptoms of intoxication include headache, dizziness, weakness, incoordination, agitation, and confusion, which can progress to coma. Seizures may occur. With the metabolism of methanol to formic acid, many other toxic effects are seen, some of which are lethal. Survivors may be blind or neurologically impaired.
Preparation of patient	None needed
Indications	Clinical suspicion of methanol ingestion
Reference range	Not applicable. The assay will not detect a level <5 mg/dL.
Critical value(s)	Toxicity usually at levels >20 mg/dL (>6.24 mmol/L). In susceptible individuals, lower concentrations in plasma may be associated with toxicity.
Increased levels	• Accidental ingestion (e.g., by a child) • Intentional overdose • Abuse in place of ethanol
Decreased levels	Not applicable
Interfering factors	The plasma level may be below the assay's limit of detection even though the patient shows signs of toxicity.
Cross-references	Methanol Poisoning Osmolality (Serum and Urine)

Multiple sleep latency test (MSLT); maintenance of wakefulness test (MWT)

Type of test	Neurophysiology
Explanation of test	The MSLT provides an index of the patient's degree of daytime sleepiness. The test is performed in the laboratory. The patient is given the opportunity to nap at least four times at 2-hour intervals throughout the day and is instructed not to resist the urge to fall asleep. Electroencephalography, electro-oculography, electromyography, and electrocardiography are used to determine times of sleep onset and offset as well as rapid eye movement (REM) sleep and to monitor heart rate and rhythm.
	The MWT provides an index of the patient's ability to stay awake during the daytime. In this test, the patient is instructed to resist the urge to fall asleep; otherwise, the protocol is much like the MSLT.
Relevance to psychiatry and behavioral science	Daytime somnolence is frequently reported in certain subsets of the population of neuropsychiatric patients, including those with Parkinson's disease, Alzheimer's disease, chronic fatigue syndrome, fibromyalgia or other chronic pain syndromes, and depression. It also plagues those treated with highly sedating medications such as anticonvulsants and antipsychotics. It is the hallmark of primary hypersomnia (narcolepsy), which is the main indication for the MSLT.
Preparation of patient	The MSLT and the MWT are often performed in the laboratory on the day after an overnight polysomnographic study. The patient should be instructed to avoid caffeine after polysomnography, until the MSLT/MWT is completed.
Indications	• Evaluating daytime hypersomnolence
	• Confirming the clinical diagnoses of primary hypersomnia and narcolepsy without cataplexy
	• Determining the effectiveness of treatment for daytime hypersomnolence
Reference range	MSLT: Average sleep latency is 10–20 minutes
	MWT: Average sleep latency on the 40-minute test is 35 minutes; average sleep latency on the 20-minute test is 18 minutes.
Critical value(s)	None
Positive test	MSLT: Average sleep onset is <8 minutes with or without sleep-onset REM periods (SOREMPs).
	If >2 SOREMPs are observed, narcolepsy without cataplexy can be diagnosed.

Multiple sleep latency test (MSLT); maintenance of wakefulness test (MWT) *(continued)*

Interfering factors	Sleep deprivation, which affects some individuals attempting to sleep in the artificial conditions of the laboratory, interferes with both the MSLT and the MWT. Environmental factors such as light, temperature, and noise affect test validity. Caffeine or other stimulants and sedative-hypnotic medications taken before the testing may invalidate results.
Cross-reference	Polysomnography (PSG)

Rack M, Davis J, Roffwarg HP, et al: The multiple sleep latency test in the diagnosis of narcolepsy. Am J Psychiatry 162:2198–2199, author reply 2199, 2005

Sullivan SS, Kushida CA: Multiple sleep latency test and maintenance of wakefulness test. Chest 134(4):854–861, 2008

Osmolality (serum and urine)	
Type of test	Blood, urine
Explanation of test	*Osmolality* is a measure of the concentration of particulates in serum or urine per *kilogram* of water. (A related variable—*osmolarity*—measures the concentration per *liter* of water.) Osmolality is used to evaluate fluid and electrolyte balance, to determine the cause of increased or decreased urine output, to investigate abnormal levels of sodium, and to detect the presence of ingested toxins such as methanol or acetylsalicylic acid. Serum and urine osmolality are most often measured at the same time so that results can be correctly interpreted.
	Under normal conditions, the body maintains osmolality within a certain range through secretion of antidiuretic hormone (ADH) by the posterior pituitary, under the control of the hypothalamus. When osmolality increases, ADH is secreted, signaling the kidneys to conserve water. This results in a more concentrated urine and a more dilute plasma. When osmolality decreases, ADH secretion is suppressed, signaling the kidneys to produce a more dilute urine (see Figure 5 in Appendix).
	Serum osmolality is mostly a reflection of sodium concentration, whereas urine osmolality is mostly a measure of waste products (urea and creatinine). Under pathological conditions, serum osmolality can also reflect glucose levels (in hyperglycemia) or blood urea levels (in renal failure).
	Serum osmolality aids in the evaluation of hyponatremia, which may be secondary to urinary sodium losses or to increased fluid in circulation (e.g., from polydipsia, water retention, inability of the kidneys to produce a dilute urine, or high glucose levels). Another application of serum osmolality is to compare it with a calculation of predicted osmolality based on measurements of the major solutes (sodium, glucose, blood urea nitrogen [BUN]), a difference termed the *osmolal gap*. This gap indicates the presence of additional osmotically active substances such as ethanol, methanol, or ethylene glycol in the blood. Ethanol is the most common cause, with the gap roughly equal to the ethanol concentration in milligrams per deciliter divided by 4.6.

Osmolality (serum and urine) *(continued)*

Relevance to psychiatry and behavioral science	A number of psychiatric and neurological conditions are associated with derangements in osmolality. Acute osmolality changes may cause delirium, or coma in extreme cases. Causes include dehydration, hyperglycemia, alcohol withdrawal, and traumatic brain injury, among others. Subacute or chronic changes can be caused by medications (e.g., diabetes insipidus in patients treated with lithium, or syndrome of inappropriate antidiuretic hormone secretion [SIADH] in patients treated with antidepressants, antipsychotics, opioids, or carbamazepine), psychogenic polydipsia, tuberculosis, subdural hematoma, hydrocephalus, AIDS, and multiple sclerosis, among other conditions.
Preparation of patient	None needed
Indications	• Determining the cause of hyponatremia • Assessing fluid and electrolyte balance • Determining the cause of abnormal urine output • Evaluating suspected SIADH, diabetes insipidus, or psychogenic polydipsia • Detecting ingested toxins such as methanol, ethylene glycol, or acetylsalicylic acid
Reference range	*Serum osmolality* Children and adults ≤60 years: 275–295 mOsm/kg H_2O Adults >60 years: 280–301 mOsm/kg H_2O *Urine osmolality* Spot urine sample: 50–1,200 mOsm/kg H_2O, depending on fluid intake 24-hour urine sample: 300–900 mOsm/kg H_2O The normal ratio of urine to serum osmolality is 3:1.
Critical value(s)	*Serum osmolality* <240 mOsm/kg H_2O >320 mOsm/kg H_2O >360 mOsm/kg H_2O: Respiratory arrest may occur.
Increased levels	*Serum osmolality* • Dehydration • Diabetes insipidus • Hyperglycemia (diabetic ketoacidosis or nonketotic hyperosmolar coma)

Osmolality (serum and urine) *(continued)*

Increased levels *(continued)*	*Serum osmolality* (continued)
	• Hypercalcemia
	• Cerebral lesions
	• Hypernatremic ethanol intoxication
	• Tube feeding
	• High-protein diet
	• Hypovolemic shock
	• Poisoning (e.g., methanol, ethylene glycol)
	• *Drugs:* mineralocorticoids, osmotic diuretics, insulin, mannitol, herbs, and other natural remedies
	Urine osmolality
	• Dehydration
	• Prerenal azotemia
	• Congestive heart failure
	• SIADH
	• Addison disease
	• Amyloidosis
	• Hypernatremia
	• High-protein diet
	• *Drugs:* carbamazepine, diuretics, mannitol, X-ray contrast agents, and others
Decreased levels	*Serum osmolality*
	• Overhydration
	• Primary (psychogenic) polydipsia
	• Addison disease
	• Acute renal failure
	• Panhypopituitarism
	• Postoperative states
	• SIADH

Osmolality (serum and urine) *(continued)*	
Decreased levels *(continued)*	*Urine osmolality* • Acute renal failure • Diabetes insipidus • Primary (psychogenic) polydipsia • Compulsive water drinking • Electrolyte derangement: hypokalemia, hypernatremia, or hypercalcemia
Interfering factors	Specimen hemolysis or lipemic serum influences result.
Cross-references	Polydipsia (Psychogenic) Syndrome of Inappropriate Antidiuretic Hormone Secretion (SIADH)

Oxazepam level	
Type of test	Blood
Explanation of test	Benzodiazepines are Schedule IV sedative-hypnotic drugs used to treat anxiety and insomnia. Oxazepam is a drug with a slow onset of action and a short half-life. It is not extensively metabolized in the liver. In general, levels of the drug are checked when either overdose or noncompliance is suspected or to detect use without a prescription. In the latter case, a urine drug screen is more likely to be ordered than a blood level.
Relevance to psychiatry and behavioral science	Toxicity with chronic benzodiazepine ingestion may manifest as confusion, disorientation, memory impairment, ataxia, decreased reflexes, and dysarthria. With acute overdose, the patient may exhibit somnolence, confusion, ataxia, decreased reflexes, vertigo, dysarthria, respiratory depression, and coma. More serious consequences usually involve co-ingestion of alcohol or other sedatives. If the ingestion was within 4 hours or if the patient is symptomatic, activated charcoal should be given and then repeated as needed. Administration of flumazenil does not affect oxazepam level.
Preparation of patient	None needed
Indications	• Screening for drug use • Suspicion of overdose • Signs of toxicity in a treated patient • Suspected noncompliance with prescribed therapy
Reference range	0.15–1.4 µg/mL
Critical value(s)	>2.0 µg/mL
Increased levels	• Overdose • Overuse
Decreased levels	Noncompliance
Interfering factors	None
Cross-references	Benzodiazepines Drug Screen (Toxicology Screen)

Phosphate
(also known as phosphorus)

Type of test	Blood
Explanation of test	Phosphorus is a mineral ingested from dietary sources that include meats, chicken, fish, eggs, dairy products, beans, nuts, and cereals. Its absorption in the small intestine is facilitated by vitamin D. In the body, phosphorus combines with other substances to produce both organic and inorganic phosphate compounds. Up to 85% of phosphorus binds to calcium to form bones and teeth; of the remainder, 10% resides in muscle, 1% in nerve tissue, and 1% in the blood.
	This test measures the amount of inorganic phosphate in blood. This level is regulated by changes in intestinal absorption and/or renal excretion. Phosphates have a number of important functions in the body, including acid-base balance, carbohydrate and lipid metabolism, and storage and transfer of energy. Phosphate levels are most often checked along with levels of calcium, parathyroid hormone, and vitamin D to diagnose and monitor treatment of conditions that affect both phosphate and calcium levels.
Relevance to psychiatry and behavioral science	Patients with mild to moderate phosphate deficiency may be asymptomatic. Those with severe deficiency may exhibit muscle weakness, reduced cardiac contractility, reduced platelet function, paresthesias, and confusion. Patients who are on ventilators may have difficulty weaning if phosphate deficiency is present. As severity of phosphate deficiency worsens, muscle cramps, delirium, and seizures may be seen. Alcoholism is associated with decreased phosphate levels, whereas cirrhosis is associated with increased levels. Patients who ingest large volumes of soft drinks or large amounts of prepackaged foods may develop toxic levels of phosphate.
Preparation of patient	Patient should fast for 8–12 hours before testing.
Indications	• Abnormal calcium result • Symptoms of an abnormal calcium level • Workup and monitoring of kidney disease • Workup and monitoring of gastrointestinal disease
Reference range	Children 2–12 years: 4.5–5.5 mg/dL (1.45–1.78 mmol/L) Adults ≤60 years: 2.7–4.5 mg/dL (0.87–1.45 mmol/L) Females >60 years: 2.8–4.1 mg/dL (0.90–1.30 mmol/L) Males >60 years: 2.3–3.7 mg/dL (0.74–1.20 mmol/L)
Critical value(s)	<1.0 mg/dL (<0.32 mmol/L)

Phosphate (also known as phosphorus) *(continued)*	
Increased levels	• Kidney failure • Hypoparathyroidism • Hypocalcemia • Excessive vitamin D intake • Liver disease and cirrhosis • Pulmonary embolism • Addison disease • Acromegaly • Healing fractures • Osteolytic bone tumors and metastases • Increased intake (e.g., phosphate supplements, overconsumption of phosphate-containing soda drinks) • Use of laxatives or enemas with high phosphate content is associated with significant phosphate elevation starting 2–3 hours after exposure and lasting up to 6 hours.
Decreased levels	• Hyperparathyroidism • Hypercalcemia • Malnutrition • Malabsorption • Vomiting and severe diarrhea • Acid/base imbalance • Overuse of diuretics • Alcoholism and liver disease • Vitamin D deficiency (rickets and/or osteomalacia) • Growth hormone deficiency • Continuous intravenous administration of glucose • Salicylate poisoning • Sepsis

Phosphate
(also known as phosphorus) (continued)

Interfering factors	Phosphate levels show diurnal fluctuation, with highest levels in late morning and lowest in evening. Environmental factors that affect phosphate levels include ingestion of carbohydrates, use of phosphate-binding antacids, and normal fluctuations in renal function as well as growth hormone and insulin secretion. Both menopause and bed rest are associated with increased levels, and menstruation with decreased levels. Falsely elevated phosphate levels may be measured if serum or plasma is not separated from erythrocytes within 1 hour after blood is drawn. Falsely elevated phosphate levels may also occur with the use of anabolic steroids, beta-blockers, ethanol, diuretics, growth hormone, and vitamin D. Falsely decreased levels may occur with the use of aluminum-containing antacids, acetazolamide, estrogens, mannitol, albuterol, carbamazepine, phenytoin, epinephrine, or phenothiazines, among other drugs.
Cross-references	Anorexia Nervosa
	Calcium (Ca^{++})
	Eating Disorders
	Magnesium (Mg^{++})
	Renal Function Panel
	Vitamin D

Platelet count

Type of test	Blood
Explanation of test	Platelets or thrombocytes are disc-shaped cells that develop in the bone marrow and spend most of their 1-week life span in the circulation. Platelets are needed for hemostasis, vasoconstriction, and small-vessel maintenance (plugging leaks in vessels). The number and size (volume) of platelets are both reported as part of the complete blood count. An insufficient number of platelets is associated with spontaneous bleeding and easy bruising. The mean platelet volume (MPV) is an indicator of the average age of platelets; newly formed platelets are larger than old platelets. *Thrombocytosis* refers to an increased number of platelets, while *thrombocytopenia* refers to a decreased number of platelets.
Relevance to psychiatry and behavioral science	Numerous psychotropic drugs are associated with changes in platelet count. Thrombocytopenia is associated with various antidepressants (all classes), antipsychotics (conventional and atypical), anticonvulsants, prescribed stimulants, acetylcholinesterase inhibitors, commonly used analgesics (aspirin, acetaminophen, codeine, ibuprofen, and others), beta-blockers, and vaccines. Thrombocytosis is associated with amoxapine, clozapine, danazol, donepezil, steroids, immune globulin, lithium, megestrol, metoprolol, paroxetine, propranolol, venlafaxine, and zidovudine, among many other drugs.
Preparation of patient	None needed
Indications	• Evaluating bleeding disorders • Monitoring bone marrow failure • Abnormal estimated platelet count on a blood smear • A component of the coagulation profile
Reference range	Adults: 140–400×10^3/mm^3 or 140–400×10^9/L Lower limit of normal may be lower for those of African or Afro-Caribbean ancestry.
Critical value(s)	<20×10^3/mm^3 or <20×10^9/L is associated with spontaneous bleeding (>50×10^3/mm^3 usually is not). >1,000×10^3/mm^3 is associated with myeloproliferative disorders. Patients with these platelet values may have bleeding because of abnormal platelet *function*. Half of patients with an unexpected increase in platelet count have malignancy.

Platelet count *(continued)*	
Increased levels	• Essential thrombocytosis • Rapid blood regeneration (e.g., acute bleeding) • Leukemia, myeloproliferative disease • Hodgkin disease, lymphoma, other malignancies • Polycythemia vera • Splenectomy • Iron deficiency anemia • Acute infection • Acute inflammation • Rheumatoid arthritis, systemic lupus erythematosus, collagen diseases • Chronic pancreatitis, inflammatory bowel disease, tuberculosis • Renal failure • Recovery from bone marrow suppression • Numerous drugs, including psychotropics listed in "Relevance" section above
Decreased levels	• Idiopathic thrombocytopenic purpura • Various heritable syndromes • Anemia (pernicious, hemolytic, aplastic) • Thrombopoietin deficiency • Dilutional effect of a large blood transfusion • Infection (viral, bacterial, or rickettsial) • Congestive heart failure, congenital heart disease • Chemotherapy or radiation therapy • Exposure to DDT (dichlorodiphenyltrichloroethane) and other chemicals • HIV infection • Bone marrow disease (leukemia, carcinoma, myelofibrosis) • Disseminated intravascular coagulation, thrombotic thrombocytopenic purpura • Preeclampsia, eclampsia • Alcoholism, excessive alcohol ingestion

Platelet count *(continued)*	
Decreased levels *(continued)*	• Hypersplenism • Renal insufficiency • Antiplatelet antibodies • Numerous drugs, including psychotropics listed in "Relevance" section above
Interfering factors	Platelet clumps or giant platelets make automated counts inaccurate; in these cases, manual inspection will be required. Thrombocytosis may be seen at high altitudes, in winter, or after strenuous exercise, trauma, or excitement. Thrombocytopenia may be observed before monthly menstruation and during pregnancy.
Cross-reference	Complete Blood Count (CBC)

Polysomnography (PSG)

Type of test	Neurophysiology
Explanation of test	In PSG, multiple parameters are monitored and techniques performed during sleep, including electroencephalogram, eye movements (measured by electro-oculogram), electrocardiogram (ECG), electromyogram (EMG) of chin muscle, EMG of anterior tibialis muscle, respiratory effort of chest and abdomen, oral/nasal airflow, and oxygen saturation. Digital data capture has simplified the detection of sleep-related events and the scoring of sleep stages and events. As a means to reduce the cost of this procedure, ambulatory (at-home) recording modules have been developed. Although a number of disorders can be detected using PSG, the primary indication for this procedure is that of confirming the clinical diagnosis of sleep apnea. For this purpose, apnea and hypopnea events are monitored. Apnea occurs when airflow stops for more than 10 seconds. Hypopnea occurs when airflow is reduced by 50% for more than 10 seconds. The apnea-hypopnea index (AHI) is the sum of apneas and hypopneas per hour of sleep.
Relevance to psychiatry and behavioral science	PSG study can aid in diagnosing and characterizing several conditions that affect patients in psychiatric practice, including nocturnal panic attacks, sleep apnea with treatment-resistant depression, cognitive impairment with nocturnal desaturation, and various parasomnias. Results of PSG study related to the AHI can be helpful in reinforcing weight loss in patients with obstructive sleep apnea (OSA), because the AHI may significantly improve with weight loss.
Preparation of patient	The patient stays overnight in the sleep laboratory while undergoing monitoring. Video recording is also needed if the referring question relates to rapid eye movement (REM) behavior disorder. If the patient has OSA and the intention is to initiate continuous positive airway pressure (CPAP) treatment, a mask will be worn for part of the night to determine settings.
Indications	• Evaluating sleep-disordered breathing • Confirming diagnosis of restless legs syndrome • Detecting periodic limb movements of sleep • Evaluating REM behavior disorder • Confirming nocturnal seizures • Confirming nocturnal panic attacks (to exclude seizures) • Confirming other parasomnias such as sleepwalking

Polysomnography (PSG) *(continued)*	
Reference range	<ul><li>Per laboratory report, normal values for the following:<ul><li>Sleep onset and offset times (hours of sleep)</li><li>Proportion of each sleep stage</li><li>Number of arousals during sleep</li></ul></li><li>Absence of periodic leg movements or jerks</li><li>Oxygen saturation >90% (oxygen desaturation index <5 events per hour of saturation <90%)</li><li>Absence of abnormal snoring</li><li>Absence of heart rate and rhythm disturbances on ECG</li><li>AHI ≤ 5 apneas/hypopneas per hour (≤10 per hour after age 60 years) not consistent with OSA</li></ul>
Critical value(s)	Mild sleep apnea: AHI>5 Moderate sleep apnea: AHI 15–30 Severe sleep apnea: AHI>30
Abnormal test	<ul><li>Apneas (significant number)</li><li>Hypopneas (significant number)</li><li>Desaturation<90%</li><li>Disrupted sleep architecture</li><li>Abnormal leg movements</li><li>Abnormal behaviors</li></ul>
Interfering factors	Caffeine or stimulants and sedative-hypnotic medications taken before testing can significantly interfere with test results.
Cross-references	None

Flemons WW: Clinical practice. Obstructive sleep apnea. N Engl J Med 347(7):498–504, 2002

Positron emission tomography (PET): brain	
Type of test	Imaging, nuclear medicine
Explanation of test	In PET scanning, a gamma ray–emitting isotope (radionuclide) is coupled with a biologically active molecule or drug of interest, and the concentration of radionuclide activity is subsequently mapped to show the location of the coupled molecule/drug. If the coupled molecule is fluorodeoxyglucose (FDG), the scan yields information about tissue metabolic activity. In fact, a number of different isotopes are available for use with PET, including ^{15}O, ^{13}N, and ^{11}C, but ^{18}F coupled with glucose (FDG) is most commonly employed in clinical scanning. ^{18}F has a long enough half-life that it is possible to produce the isotope at an off-site facility. In addition, it is less critical that the patient's mental state or activity be standardized with this isotope than with isotopes with very short half-lives such as ^{15}O. Other molecules can be appended in place of glucose. One such example is florbetapir (^{18}F-AV-45), which binds to beta-amyloid protein to allow brain amyloid deposits in patients with suspected Alzheimer's disease to be visualized in vivo. This compound has a long enough half-life that it can be express-shipped between states for use. PET scanning in clinical and research settings usually also includes anatomical imaging in the form of computed tomography or magnetic resonance imaging to co-register metabolic findings with anatomy.
Relevance to psychiatry and behavioral science	FDG-PET is in current use for the differential diagnosis of dementia when history, physical exam, and other tests are inconclusive. Amyloid imaging is in current use for patients being evaluated for dementia or mild cognitive impairment. In Parkinson disease, either PET or single-photon emission computed tomography (dopamine transporter scanning) can be helpful.
Preparation of patient	Diuretics should be held before the test, and the patient should avoid ingesting large amounts of fluid or caffeine-containing beverages because it will be necessary for him or her to remain immobile in the scanner for 30 minutes. The entire procedure takes 60–90 minutes because of the need to wait for uptake of the injected compound before scanning. Patients should be instructed to eat, and those on insulin should be instructed to take their medication as usual.
Indications	• Differential diagnosis of dementia subtypes • Presurgical evaluation for epilepsy • Differentiation of benign from malignant tumors • Aiding in the diagnosis of Parkinson's disease • Research protocols

Positron emission tomography (PET): brain *(continued)*	
Normal result	Requires individual interpretation according to the study protocol; in general, no abnormal accumulation of radiotracer and no unexpected gaps in the visualization of the tracer to suggest hypometabolism
Abnormal result	• Temporoparietal hypometabolism in Alzheimer's disease; often more marked in one hemisphere • Frontal or frontotemporal hypometabolism in frontal lobe dementia • Increased uptake in vascular tumor • Abnormal uptake in seizure focus, dependent on time since seizure
Interfering factors	Hypoglycemia can affect glucose metabolism as imaged by FDG-PET. Movement of the patient of more than 1 cm can result in motion artifact.
Cross-references	None

Herholz K, Carter SF, Jones M: Positron emission tomography imaging in dementia. Br J Radiol 80(Spec No 2):S160–S167, 2007

Mosconi L, Tsui WH, Herholz K, et al: Multicenter standardized 18F-FDG PET diagnosis of mild cognitive impairment, Alzheimer's disease, and other dementias. J Nucl Med 49(3):390–398, 2008

Potassium (K⁺)

Type of test	Blood
Explanation of test	Potassium is an electrolyte present in all body fluids. It is concentrated inside cells, where it functions to regulate water and acid-base balance, participate in nerve conduction, and stimulate contraction of muscle cells. Along with calcium and magnesium, potassium controls cardiac output (heart rate and force of contraction). Potassium is taken in from dietary sources and excreted primarily through the glomeruli of the kidneys. Mildly decreased potassium levels are common, particularly among patients treated with diuretic medications. Increased potassium levels result primarily from cellular injury (when potassium is released into the circulation) or reduced renal function.
Relevance to psychiatry and behavioral science	Severe hyperkalemia (increased potassium level) or hypokalemia (decreased potassium level) can be life-threatening conditions requiring urgent intervention. Potassium may be increased with lithium treatment, with succinylcholine used for electroconvulsive therapy, or in acute starvation (as in anorexia nervosa). Potassium may be decreased in chronic starvation, bulimia, psychogenic vomiting, anabolic steroid abuse, or alcoholism. Patients with megaloblastic anemia treated with vitamin B_{12} or folate may become potassium depleted and require routine replacement.
Preparation of patient	The patient should avoid vigorous exercise on the day of testing, before blood is drawn.
Indications	• Admission laboratory testing • Altered mental status • Routine component of health screening • Monitoring patients on diuretic medications • Signs/symptoms of cardiac conduction disturbance • Kidney disease • Monitoring patients on dialysis or intravenous (IV) therapy
Reference range	3.5–5.1 mEq/L (3.5–5.1 mmol/L)
Critical value(s)	<2 mEq/L associated with ventricular fibrillation >7 mEq/L associated with muscular irritability (including myocardium, with peaked T waves)

Potassium (K⁺) *(continued)*	
Increased levels	• Renal failure • Dehydration • Renal obstruction • Cellular injury (burns, trauma, surgery, tissue ischemia, chemotherapy) • Intravascular hemolysis • Metabolic acidosis, diabetic ketoacidosis • Severe acute starvation (anorexia nervosa) • Status epilepticus • Malignant hyperthermia • Addison disease • Rapid potassium infusion • Acquired hyperkalemia (e.g., in systemic lupus erythematosus or sickle cell disease) • *Drugs:* nonsteroidal anti-inflammatory drugs, potassium-sparing diuretics, angiotensin-converting enzyme (ACE) inhibitors, and beta-blockers
Decreased levels	• Chronic starvation • Prolonged intravenous hydration without potassium replacement • Prolonged vomiting, diarrhea, or fluid loss from an intestinal fistula • Excessive loss of potassium in urine • Loss from draining wounds • Chronic alcoholism • Megaloblastic anemia treated with vitamin B_{12} or folate • Cystic fibrosis • *Drugs:* corticosteroids, β-adrenergic agonists such as isoproterenol, β-adrenergic antagonists such as clonidine, antibiotics such as gentamicin and carbenicillin, and the antifungal agent amphotericin B

Potassium (K⁺) *(continued)*

Interfering factors	Improper specimen handling is an important cause of spurious potassium elevation in outpatient settings, where blood has to be transported to the laboratory. Regardless of the setting, specimen hemolysis can be problematic. Use of a tourniquet and/or pumping the hand before drawing blood can elevate the potassium level by 20%. Patients with elevated white blood cell and platelet counts may also have spurious elevation of the potassium level. Some diurnal variation is seen in potassium levels, with values being 0.2–0.4 mEq/L higher in the afternoon and evening. Vigorous exercise can transiently increase potassium levels by 50%, and this effect is enhanced by beta-blockers.
Cross-references	Anorexia Nervosa
	Eating Disorders

Dørup I: Magnesium and potassium deficiency. Its diagnosis, occurrence and treatment in diuretic therapy and its consequences for growth, protein synthesis and growth factors. Acta Physiol Scand Suppl 618:1–55, 1994

Saxena K: Clinical features and management of poisoning due to potassium chloride. Med Toxicol Adverse Drug Exp 4(6):429–443, 1989

Prealbumin	
Type of test	Blood
Explanation of test	Prealbumin is a protein synthesized in the liver that serves as an indicator of nutritional function and liver disease. It is superior to albumin for this purpose because it has a shorter half-life (2–4 days compared with albumin's 22 days), so it becomes abnormal more quickly with undernutrition. This condition occurs commonly in hospitalized patients who are postoperative or critically ill and can lead to serious medical complications.
Relevance to psychiatry and behavioral science	Low prealbumin levels may be found in patients with AIDS, cancer, anorexia, and failure to thrive. Low prealbumin is a risk factor for the development of delirium.
Preparation of patient	None needed
Indications	• Presurgical evaluation • Evaluating nutritional status in hospitalized patients • Workup for anorexia nervosa and other eating disorders • Diagnosing malnutrition in patients with AIDS • Patients with signs/symptoms of malnutrition • Monitoring the effects of treatment for malnutrition • Monitoring patients on hemodialysis or parenteral feeding
Reference range	Adults: 18–45 mg/dL (180–450 mg/L)
Critical value(s)	None
Increased levels	• High-dose steroids • Adrenal gland hyperfunction • High-dose nonsteroidal anti-inflammatory drugs • Hodgkin disease • Shigellosis • False elevations with renal failure
Decreased levels	• Undernutrition or malnutrition (protein-calorie) • Severe or chronic disease (e.g., cancer) • Hyperthyroidism • Liver disease • Cystic fibrosis • Diabetes mellitus • Serious infections

Prealbumin *(continued)*	
Decreased levels *(continued)*	• Certain digestive disorders (protein-losing) • Peritoneal dialysis • With inflammation in the context of undernutrition, prealbumin levels can fall quickly to very low levels. • *Drugs:* amiodarone, estrogens (including oral contraceptives)
Interfering factors	Prealbumin is a negative acute-phase reactant, so low levels can be found despite adequate nutritional stores; it may be necessary to measure simultaneously an inflammatory marker such as C-reactive protein.
Cross-references	Anorexia Nervosa Eating Disorders HIV/AIDS Hyperthyroidism

Beck FK, Rosenthal TC: Prealbumin: a marker for nutritional evaluation. Am Fam Physician 65(8):1575–1578, 2002

Prolactin (PRL)	
Type of test	Blood
Explanation of test	PRL is a protein hormone produced in the pituitary gland, central nervous system (CNS), and other tissues. Its primary action is to promote lactation in response to a suckling stimulus, but it has other roles in parental behaviors and maintenance of homeostasis. It is found in widespread areas of the brain, including the hypothalamus, hippocampus, cerebral cortex, amygdala, and caudate-putamen. PRL secretion is under inhibitory control by dopamine from the hypothalamus as well as other factors in the CNS and elsewhere.
Relevance to psychiatry and behavioral science	Dopamine receptor antagonists such as antipsychotics can cause significant PRL elevations, with consequent amenorrhea, galactorrhea, erectile dysfunction, and infertility. First-generation antipsychotics and risperidone cause the greatest PRL elevations, while aripiprazole and ziprasidone are thought to be relatively free of this effect. *Seizure detection:* During an epileptic seizure, ictal activity in mesial temporal structures is thought to propagate to the hypothalamus and alter PRL release. A PRL level that is twice the baseline value or greater can help distinguish a generalized tonic-clonic seizure or complex partial seizure from a nonepileptic seizure. PRL-secreting adenomas are pituitary tumors that may be large enough to exert mass effects, causing symptoms such as headaches, cranial nerve palsies, and visual changes. Cocaine withdrawal may cause PRL elevation. Elevated PRL levels have been associated with psychosomatic conditions such as pseudopregnancy.
Preparation of patient	For routine testing, the blood sample is drawn several hours after awakening in the morning, following 30 minutes of quiet rest. For use in diagnosing epileptic seizures, the test sample is drawn 10–20 minutes after the suspected ictal event, and the baseline sample is drawn more than 6 hours after the event.
Indications	• Identifying or excluding PRL elevation as a cause of clinical symptoms in antipsychotic-treated patients • Providing laboratory confirmation of generalized tonic-clonic seizure or complex partial seizure • Workup for suspected PRL elevation (symptoms of galactorrhea, headaches, visual disturbances, and menstrual irregularities)

Prolactin (PRL) *(continued)*	
Indications *(continued)*	• Diagnosing cause of infertility in women, and infertility and erectile dysfunction in men • Follow-up of low testosterone level • Evaluating anterior pituitary function (with other hormones) • Monitoring effectiveness of treatment for PRL-secreting tumors (prolactinomas) • Detecting recurrence of prolactinomas
Reference range	Nonpregnant females: 4–23 ng/mL Pregnant females: 34–386 ng/mL Adult males: 3–15 ng/mL Children: 3.2–20 ng/mL *Note:* 1 ng/mL=1 µg/L
Critical value(s)	A level of >200 ng/mL (>200 µg/L) in a nonlactating female indicates the presence of a prolactinoma. A normal level does not rule out a prolactinoma.
Increased levels	• Prolactinoma • Pregnancy • Nursing • Hypothalamic disease • Hypothyroidism • Kidney disease • Other pituitary tumors and diseases • Polycystic ovary syndrome • Recent seizure • Cocaine withdrawal • *Drugs:* antipsychotics, other dopamine-blocking drugs (e.g., prochlorperazine, metoclopramide), tricyclic antidepressants, ramelteon, and estrogen

Prolactin (PRL) *(continued)*	
Decreased levels	• Hypopituitarism • *Drugs:* dopamine, levodopa, and ergot alkaloid derivatives
Interfering factors	Stress from illness, trauma, or needle phobia can cause moderate increases in PRL levels. Time of sample can affect results: levels rise during sleep and peak in the morning hours. PRL can form macromolecular complexes with immunoglobulin G, leading to false-positive test results.
Cross-references	None

Chen DK, So YT, Fisher RS; Therapeutics and Technology Assessment Subcommittee of the American Academy of Neurology: Use of serum prolactin in diagnosing epileptic seizures: report of the Therapeutics and Technology Assessment Subcommittee of the American Academy of Neurology. Neurology 65(5):668–675, 2005

Freeman ME, Kanyicska B, Lerant A, Nagy G: Prolactin: structure, function, and regulation of secretion. Physiol Rev 80(4):1523–1631, 2000

Misra M, Papakostas GI, Klibanski A: Effects of psychiatric disorders and psychotropic medications on prolactin and bone metabolism. J Clin Psychiatry 65:1607–1618, quiz 1590, 1760–1761, 2004

Protein	
Type of test	Blood
Explanation of test	Proteins have critical roles in the body as enzymes, hormones, and transporters and as constituents of cells, tissues, and organs. Two classes of proteins are measured in blood: albumins and globulins. Albumin, which represents 60% of total protein, functions to maintain colloidal osmotic pressure within the vasculature and to transport drugs, hormones, and enzymes. Albumin is produced in the liver, and its level can be dramatically reduced by liver disease such as cirrhosis. The serum albumin level can also be reduced in kidney disease, when the nephron is no longer able to prevent loss of albumin in the urine. Globulins include antibodies, enzymes, and other essential proteins. Although measurement of total protein aids in the evaluation of nutritional status and can be helpful in screening for liver or kidney disease, it is actually more useful to know which component—albumin or globulin—is increased.
Relevance to psychiatry and behavioral science	Total protein may be low in anorexia nervosa, failure to thrive in elderly patients, alcoholism, liver disease, and postoperative patients. Low protein values are frequently encountered among patients on medical/surgical units in the general hospital and represent a risk factor for the development of delirium. It is a commonly held misconception that a low protein level and correspondingly low protein binding of drugs would result in increased drug action. In fact, reduced protein binding of drugs has little clinical effect, even among elderly patients. Unbound drug is available not only for distribution to the target organ but also for metabolism and excretion. What lowered protein binding does affect is the interpretation of laboratory measurement of total drug concentration; it is of potential concern that the patient might develop symptoms of toxicity at apparently therapeutic drug levels when protein levels are low.
Preparation of patient	None needed
Indications	• A component of the comprehensive metabolic panel • Evaluating nutritional status • Workup of signs/symptoms of liver or kidney disease • Evaluating edema
Reference range	Total protein: 6.0–8.0 g/dL (60–80 g/L) Albumin: 3.8–5.0 g/dL (38–50 g/L)
Critical value(s)	None

Protein *(continued)*	
Increased levels	• Multiple myeloma, other gammopathies • Waldenström macroglobulinemia • Granulomatous diseases such as sarcoidosis • Collagen vascular diseases such as systemic lupus erythematosus and rheumatoid arthritis • Chronic inflammatory states • Chronic infections • Dehydration (pseudohypoproteinemia)
Decreased levels	• Malnutrition • Malabsorption (celiac disease, inflammatory bowel disease) • Chronic or severe diarrhea • Postoperative state • Liver disease • Alcoholism • Kidney disease • Burns, severe skin diseases • Protein-losing enteropathy or uropathy • Severe hemorrhage, with volume replacement • Heart failure • Hypothyroidism • Prolonged immobilization • Third trimester of pregnancy
Interfering factors	Spurious elevation in protein level can be caused by prolonged tourniquet application or use of drugs such as anabolic steroids, androgens, corticosteroids, dextran, growth hormone, insulin, phenazopyridine, or progesterone. Spurious decrease in protein level can be caused by sampling proximal to an intravenous catheter, massive infusion of crystalloid solution, or use of drugs such as ammonium ion, estrogen, or oral contraceptives.
Cross-references	Albumin Anorexia Nervosa; Eating Disorders Comprehensive Metabolic Panel (CMP)

Fuhrman MP, Charney P, Mueller CM: Hepatic proteins and nutrition assessment. J Am Diet Assoc 104(8):1258–1264, 2004

Jacobson SA, Pies RW, Katz IR: Clinical Manual of Geriatric Psychopharmacology. Washington, DC, American Psychiatric Publishing, 2007

Pyridoxine (vitamin B_6)

Type of test	Blood
Explanation of test	Of the different forms of the B vitamin pyridoxine, the most important in plasma is pyridoxal phosphate, which is required for myelin formation and synthesis of the neurotransmitters serotonin and norepinephrine, among other functions. Pyridoxine deficiency usually occurs in the context of other nutrient deficiencies. Sources of pyridoxine in the diet include beans, nuts, meats, fish, certain vegetables (e.g., carrots, spinach), dairy products, and enriched foods such as cereals and flour. Chronic supplementation may cause an overdose neuropathy syndrome.
Relevance to psychiatry and behavioral science	Mild deficiency of pyridoxine is fairly common. Clinical pyridoxine deficiency in adults is associated with anemia, seborrhea, cheilosis, glossitis, and peripheral neuropathy. In children, neuropsychiatric symptoms are also seen, including the following: • Irritability • Weakness • Depression • Dizziness • Seizures • Confusional states (with amnesia, disorientation, and other cortical impairments) Diarrhea and failure to thrive may also be seen in affected children.
Preparation of patient	None needed
Indications	Clinical suspicion of pyridoxine deficiency
Reference range	5–50 ng/mL (20–202 nmol/L)
Critical value(s)	Deficiency: <5 ng/mL (<20 nmol/L)
Increased levels	Excessive supplementation
Decreased levels	• Alcoholism • Cirrhosis • Hyperthyroidism • Malnutrition, eating disorders • Malabsorption • Congestive heart failure

Pyridoxine (vitamin B$_6$) *(continued)*	
Decreased levels *(continued)*	• Drugs that antagonize pyridoxine or cause increased requirements: tricyclic antidepressants, anticonvulsants, cycloserine, disulfiram, isoniazid (INH), penicillamine, hydralazine, estrogens (including birth control pills), and theophylline
Interfering factors	Levels decrease with age, although age norms are not available. Specimen handling affects results; specimen must be received in the lab within 30 minutes of collection. Prolonged light exposure invalidates results.
Cross-references	None

Red blood cell count (RBC)

Type of test	Blood
Explanation of test	Red blood cells are the most numerous blood cells in the circulation. They are formed in bone marrow and have a life cycle of about 120 days. These cells function to carry hemoglobin bound to oxygen from the lungs to tissues, and carbon dioxide from the tissues to the lungs.
Relevance to psychiatry and behavioral science	Low RBC is associated with symptoms of fatigue, weakness, somnolence, anhedonia, and depression.
Preparation of patient	Fasting is not required. The patient should avoid dehydration and overhydration. Signs of severe anemia should be noted before blood is drawn. Note on requisition if patient is receiving intravenous fluids.
Indications	• Routine part of the complete blood count • Clinical suspicion of anemia or polycythemia
Reference range	Adult males: $4.5–5.5 \times 10^6/mm^3$ or $\times 10^{12}/L$ Adult females: $4.0–5.0 \times 10^6/mm^3$ or $\times 10^{12}/L$
Critical value(s)	None
Increased levels	*Primary erythrocytosis* • Polycythemia vera (a myeloproliferative disorder) • Erythremic erythrocytosis (increased red blood cell production in bone marrow) *Secondary erythrocytosis* • Renal disease • Extrarenal tumors • High altitude • Pulmonary disease • Cardiovascular disease • Alveolar hypoventilation • Hemoglobinopathy • Tobacco, carboxyhemoglobin *Relative erythrocytosis* (decreased plasma volume) • Dehydration (from vomiting, diarrhea) • Gaisböck syndrome

Red blood cell count (RBC) *(continued)*	
Decreased levels	• Anemia secondary to cell destruction, blood loss, or dietary insufficiency of iron or vitamins essential to RBC production • Lymphoma, leukemia, or multiple myeloma • Hemorrhage • Chronic disease or infection • Lupus, Addison disease, rheumatic fever, and other diseases
Interfering factors	Blood collection technique significantly affects results. If the patient is recumbent during phlebotomy, the result is 5% lower. The result is elevated with prolonged venous stasis during phlebotomy. The lavender tube must be three-fourths full or results will be invalid. A clotted sample will yield invalid results. In addition, dehydration, stress, and high altitude increase the RBC, and pregnancy decreases the RBC. Many psychotropic medications can cause a spurious reduction in the RBC, including amitriptyline, amphetamines, barbiturates, bupropion, carbamazepine, chlordiazepoxide, chlorpromazine, clomipramine, clonazepam, desipramine, diphenhydramine, donepezil, fluphenazine, haloperidol, levodopa, monoamine oxidase inhibitors, meprobamate, mesoridazine, pemoline, phenobarbital, phenytoin, thioridazine, thiothixene, trazodone, and trifluoperazine.
Cross-references	Complete Blood Count (CBC) Hematocrit (Hct) Mean Corpuscular Volume (MCV)

Renal function panel	
Type of test	Blood
Explanation of tests	The panel consists of the following tests: albumin, blood urea nitrogen (BUN), calcium, total carbon dioxide, chloride, creatinine, glucose, phosphate, potassium, and sodium. Risk factors for acute renal disease include a history of trauma, sepsis, hypotension, and reaction to contrast dye. Risk factors for chronic renal disease include hypertension, diabetes, atherosclerosis, familial kidney disease, polycystic kidneys, and use of nephrotoxic drugs such as nonsteroidal anti-inflammatory drugs.
Relevance to psychiatry and behavioral science	Impaired renal function is associated with a spectrum of neuropsychiatric symptoms, ranging from fatigue and lethargy to delirium and coma. Cognitive impairment, sleep and appetite disturbances, and sexual dysfunction also have been reported. Since most psychotropic drugs are excreted at least partly by the kidneys, changes in renal function have definite pharmacokinetic effects. Lithium is eliminated only through the kidneys, such that the serum level is directly proportional to the glomerular filtration rate. Lithium and other drugs such as gabapentin can in turn affect kidney function. Lithium is associated with diabetes insipidus, and with long-term use can cause tubulointerstitial disease. The use of lithium necessitates renal function monitoring, as described in Chapter 3, "Psychotropic Medications."
Preparation of patient	None needed
Indications	• Workup for patient with risk factors for acute or chronic kidney disease • Monitoring patients with diabetes for early renal dysfunction
Reference range	See entries for individual tests.
Critical value(s)	
Increased levels	
Decreased levels	
Interfering factors	
Cross-references	Lithium See entries for individual tests.

Single-photon emission computed tomography (SPECT)

Type of test	Nuclear medicine
Explanation of test	SPECT utilizes a radiopharmaceutical such as technetium-labeled hexamethylpropyleneamine oxime (^{99m}Tc-HMPAO) to visualize blood flow to various areas of the brain. This compound crosses the blood-brain barrier, decomposes, and remains in the brain for several hours. The distribution of the compound is imaged by the SPECT camera in 3D and then represented in 2D images. SPECT is less costly than positron emission tomography (PET), and the equipment is more universally available in medical settings. It is also not as problematic for patients with claustrophobia, because the camera is less confining than the PET scanner. The primary reason that PET is preferred in neuropsychiatric research settings has to do with spatial resolution; resolution with SPECT is on the order of about 1 cm, which is too coarse for the study of many brain structures of interest. In general, the indications are similar to those of PET, although less well validated. Where PET shows hypometabolism, SPECT could be expected to show hypoperfusion. One controversial clinical application of SPECT has been in the diagnosis of attention-deficit/hyperactivity disorder. Like PET, SPECT is often coupled with computed tomography or magnetic resonance imaging to show anatomical landmarks.
Relevance to psychiatry and behavioral science	For uses not highly dependent on resolution of small structures, SPECT is considered equivalent to PET for diagnosis.
Preparation of patient	The patient should eat before the test and take medications as usual but should avoid drinking large amounts of liquid or caffeinated beverages because of the need to remain still for 30 minutes while the scan takes place. No other preparation is needed.
Indications	• Differential diagnosis of dementia subtypes • Presurgical evaluation for epilepsy • Differentiation of benign from malignant tumors • Diagnosing Parkinson's disease • Research protocols
Normal result	Normal blood flow patterns
Abnormal result	• Globally reduced blood flow • Regionally or focally reduced blood flow • Focally increased blood flow

Single-photon emission computed tomography (SPECT) *(continued)*	
Interfering factors	The clinical value of SPECT scanning depends to a large extent on the expertise of the interpreter. One commonly seen false-positive finding is *crossed cerebellar diaschisis*, in which reduced cerebellar blood flow is seen contralateral to the hypoperfusion associated with a lesion such as a middle cerebral artery infarct.
Cross-reference	Positron Emission Tomography (PET): Brain

Catafau AM: Brain SPECT in clinical practice, part I: perfusion. J Nucl Med 42(2):259–271, 2001
Vasile RG: Single photon emission computed tomography in psychiatry: current perspectives. Harv Rev Psychiatry 4(1):27–38, 1996

Sodium (Na⁺)

Type of test	Blood
Explanation of test	As the most abundant positively charged ion in blood, sodium has critical roles in neurotransmission and maintenance of osmotic pressure. As the principal base component of blood, it also has a major role in maintenance of acid-base balance. The sodium level reflects dietary intake less renal excretion. Sodium level is maintained primarily through the actions of aldosterone (decreases renal sodium loss), natriuretic hormone (increases renal sodium loss), and antidiuretic hormone (increases resorption of water). As free body water increases or decreases, these factors stimulate the kidney to compensate to restore sodium balance. In clinical practice, sodium levels are obtained to evaluate electrolytes, acid-base balance, water balance, water intoxication, and dehydration.
Relevance to psychiatry and behavioral science	Serum sodium abnormalities are found in a number of conditions encountered in psychiatric practice, including polydipsia, lithium-induced diabetes insipidus, the syndrome of inappropriate antidiuretic hormone secretion (SIADH), beer potomania, and hypopituitarism. In addition, psychotropic drugs associated with sodium derangements include antidepressants (selective serotonin reuptake inhibitors [SSRIs] and tricyclic antidepressants [TCAs]), carbamazepine, oxcarbazepine, lithium, phenothiazines, and opioids.
Preparation of patient	None needed
Indications	• A standard component of the basic metabolic panel and the comprehensive metabolic panel • Performed for admission workup and evaluation of delirium, seizure, and SIADH
Reference range	Adults ≤90 years: 136–145 mEq/L (136–145 mmol/L) Adults >90 years: 132–146 mEq/L (132–146 mmol/L)
Critical value(s)	<120 mEq/L or >160 mEq/L
Increased levels	• Dehydration with inadequate water intake • Excessive free water loss: excessive sweating, extensive thermal burns, diabetes insipidus, osmotic diuresis • Increased sodium intake in intravenous fluids (isotonic saline) • Decreased sodium loss: hyperaldosteronism (Cushing syndrome, Conn syndrome) • Tracheobronchitis • *Drugs:* steroids (both anabolic and corticosteroids), antibiotics, clonidine, cough medicine, laxatives, methyldopa, carbenicillin, estrogens, and oral contraceptives

Sodium (Na⁺) *(continued)*	
Decreased levels	• Water intoxication, psychogenic polydipsia • SIADH • Treatment with thiazide diuretics • Transurethral resection of the prostate with infusion of non-sodium-containing irrigants • Hypothyroidism • Hyperglycemia: sodium decreases by 1.5–3.0 mEq/L for each 100 mg/dL increase in blood glucose • Hyperlipidemia • Increased sodium loss: Addison disease, diarrhea, vomiting, sweating, burns, nasogastric suction, diuretic therapy, chronic renal insufficiency • Increased free body water: excessive sodium-free oral or intravenous intake, congestive heart failure • Third-space loss of sodium: ascites, peripheral edema, pleural effusion, loss through bowel lumen in ileus or obstruction • Sodium-deficient diet • *Drugs:* lithium, carbamazepine, fluoxetine and other SSRI antidepressants, haloperidol, diuretics, sodium-free intravenous fluids, sulfonylureas, triamterene, angiotensin-converting enzyme (ACE) inhibitors, captopril, heparin, nonsteroidal anti-inflammatory drugs, opioids, oxcarbazepine, phenothiazines, TCAs, and vasopressin
Interfering factors	Recent trauma, shock, or surgery can affect sodium values. A spurious reduction of sodium (pseudohyponatremia) can occur with indirect sodium ion-selective electrode (ISE) assays in the presence of hyperproteinemia and hyperlipidemia due to decreased water content. This effect is not seen with direct ISE assays.
Cross-references	Polydipsia (Psychogenic) Syndrome of Inappropriate Antidiuretic Hormone Secretion (SIADH)

Adrogué HJ, Madias NE: Hyponatremia. N Engl J Med 342(21):1581–1589, 2000

Lien YH, Shapiro JI: Hyponatremia: clinical diagnosis and management. Am J Med 120(8):653–658, 2007

Reynolds RM, Padfield PL, Seckl JR: Disorders of sodium balance. BMJ 332(7543):702–705, 2006

Syphilis testing:
- **Rapid Plasma Reagin (RPR)**
- **Venereal Disease Research Laboratory (VDRL)**
- **Fluorescent Treponemal Antibody Absorption (FTA-Abs)**

Type of test	• Blood • Skin scraping from a visible lesion • Cerebrospinal fluid
Explanation of test	For syphilis screening, the RPR test is used, with titers drawn if the test is reactive. The VDRL test can be used as an alternative screen, with titers drawn if the test result is positive. (The RPR is preferred, because the VDRL has a higher rate of false-positive results.) If either one of these tests is positive, treponemal testing is performed, using one of the following: • FTA-Abs • Microhemagglutination assay for antibodies to *Treponema pallidum* (MHA-TP) • Immunoglobulin M antibody detection by enzyme-linked immunosorbent assay (ELISA) If these tests are reactive (antibody positive), then syphilis is likely, and the disease should be staged and treated. For suspected cases of neurosyphilis, RPR is performed on serum, and VDRL is performed on cerebrospinal fluid. If the serum RPR is negative, but there remains a suspicion for neurosyphilis, FTA-Abs is performed on serum, since some patients with late syphilis have a false-negative RPR test. In HIV patients, the affected site is usually the central nervous system. The organism *T. pallidum* cannot be cultured in vitro. If a skin lesion is present, a scraping from the lesion may be examined by darkfield microscopy in an attempt to identify the bacterium.
Relevance to psychiatry and behavioral science	Among psychiatric patients, the risk of sexually transmitted infection (STI) is higher in those with alcohol and drug abuse or dependence, bipolar disorder, and certain personality disorders, and in those who are HIV positive. With these risks in mind, appropriate vigilance regarding STI testing can be maintained. Neurosyphilis is associated with dementia, mood disorders, and behavioral changes.
Preparation of patient	None needed

Syphilis testing:
- **Rapid Plasma Reagin (RPR)**
- **Venereal Disease Research Laboratory (VDRL)**
- **Fluorescent Treponemal Antibody Absorption (FTA-Abs)** *(continued)*

Indications	• Chancre, skin rash, or other signs of syphilis • Screening in a patient with another STI such as gonorrhea • Screening in patients with newly diagnosed HIV infection • Screening for syphilis in pregnancy • Screening for syphilis to obtain a marriage license (required in many states)
Reference range	Negative or nonreactive
Positive test	Reactive RPR (VDRL) and positive treponemal testing
Negative test	Nonreactive RPR (VDRL) and negative treponemal testing
Interfering factors	False-positive RPR or VDRL results may occur in the presence of HIV disease, herpes simplex virus, primary antiphospholipid syndrome, malaria, intravenous drug use, systemic lupus erythematosus, rheumatoid arthritis, pregnancy, Hansen disease, or other treponemal diseases. False-positive FTA-Abs results may occur in the presence of autoimmune disease, Hansen disease, febrile illness, advanced age, Lyme disease, or other treponemal diseases.
Cross-references	None

Clyne B, Jerrard DA: Syphilis testing. J Emerg Med 18(3):361–367, 2000
Young H: Guidelines for serological testing for syphilis. Sex Transm Infect 76(5):403–405, 2000

Temazepam level

Type of test	Blood
Explanation of test	Benzodiazepines are Schedule IV sedative-hypnotic drugs used to treat anxiety and insomnia. Temazepam is a drug with a slow onset of action and a half-life of up to 2 days. It is not extensively metabolized in the liver. In general, levels are checked when either overdose or noncompliance is suspected or to detect use without a prescription.
Relevance to psychiatry and behavioral science	Toxicity with chronic benzodiazepine ingestion may manifest as confusion, disorientation, memory impairment, ataxia, decreased reflexes, and dysarthria. With acute overdose, the patient may exhibit somnolence, confusion, ataxia, decreased reflexes, vertigo, dysarthria, respiratory depression, and coma. More serious consequences usually involve co-ingestion of alcohol or other sedatives. If the ingestion was within 4 hours or if the patient is symptomatic, activated charcoal should be given and then repeated as needed. Administration of flumazenil does not affect the temazepam level.
Preparation of patient	None needed
Indications	• Screening for drug use • Suspicion of overdose • Signs of toxicity in a treated patient • Suspected noncompliance with prescribed therapy
Reference range	0.4–0.9 µg/mL
Critical value(s)	Levels above reference
Increased levels	• Overdose • Overuse
Decreased levels	Noncompliance
Interfering factors	None
Cross-references	Benzodiazepines Drug Screen (Toxicology Screen)

Thiamine (vitamin B₁)	
Type of test	Blood
Explanation of test	Thiamine is an essential coenzyme in several biochemical pathways. It plays a role in cognitive function, blood formation, circulation, carbohydrate metabolism, maintenance of muscle tone, and other processes. It acts as an antioxidant to protect the body from the degenerative effects of aging, smoking, and alcohol consumption. Thiamine stores in the body are limited. With inadequate dietary intake, thiamine deficiency can occur in as little as 10 days, with severe deficiency developing within 21 days. One test for measuring the adequacy of thiamine levels in the blood is the measurement of red blood cell (RBC) transketolase activity before and after the addition of thiamine pyrophosphate to the sample. If the difference in activity is >25%, then thiamine deficiency is confirmed. A difference of 15%–24% signals marginal thiamine deficiency. It is also possible to measure the primary active form of thiamine (thiamine diphosphate [TDP]) in whole blood using high-performance liquid chromatography, and this is now the preferred assay.
Relevance to psychiatry and behavioral science	Thiamine deficiency is underdiagnosed in children as well as adults, particularly those with alcoholism or AIDS. Other patients at risk include those with eating disorders and elderly patients treated with diuretics. Thiamine requirements are directly related to caloric intake, particularly carbohydrate intake. When a patient suspected to have thiamine deficiency presents to the emergency department, thiamine should be replaced before glucose to prevent precipitation of Wernicke encephalopathy in a marginally deficient patient. A mnemonic for the correct order of therapy is *Thank God I was given thiamine before glucose!* Thiamine is essential for normal cognition, learning, appetite, and growth. Other biological effects are described below. Neuropsychiatric signs of thiamine deficiency include Wernicke-Korsakoff syndrome, sensorimotor dysfunction, nystagmus, ophthalmoplegia, ataxia, confusion, and coma. The deficiency syndrome can be fatal. In patients who survive and are treated, impaired memory and other cognitive functions may persist after treatment.
Preparation of patient	The patient should fast overnight and should abstain from alcohol for 24 hours before the test.
Indications	• Suspected thiamine deficiency in a patient at risk • Cardiac, neurological, or constitutional signs consistent with thiamine deficiency

Thiamine (vitamin B₁) *(continued)*	
Reference range	Whole blood 275–675 ng/g
	Serum 0.32 ± 0.11 µg/dL
	RBC (thiamine pyrophosphate) 4.5–10.3 µg/dL
Critical value(s)	None
Increased levels	Toxicity is seen only with extremes of parenteral dosing.
Decreased levels	• Alcoholism, with or without liver disease
	• Starvation
	• Excessive consumption of raw fish or tea
	• Elderly patients
	• Patients with chronic gastrointestinal problems or prolonged diarrhea
	• Cancer
	• Diabetes
	• Long-term diuretic therapy
	• Chronic illness
	• *Drugs:* barbiturates
Interfering factors	None
Cross-references	Thiamine (Vitamin B₁) Deficiency
	Wernicke-Korsakoff Syndrome

Frankenburg FR: Alcohol use, thiamine deficiency, and cognitive impairment. JAMA 299:2854, author reply 2854–2855, 2008

Gans DA: Biochemical measures of thiamine deficiency. Am J Clin Nutr 65(4):1090–1092, 1997

Thyroid function testing: free thyroxine (free T$_4$; FT$_4$)

Type of test	Blood
Explanation of test	Thyroxine (T$_4$) is a hormone produced in the thyroid gland that is secreted in response to stimulation by thyroid-stimulating hormone (TSH) from the anterior pituitary gland. The small fraction of T$_4$ that circulates in the unbound (free) form (FT$_4$) is metabolically active and has critical roles in determining the basal metabolic rate, the synthesis of proteins, the release of calcium from bone, and the metabolism of lipids, carbohydrates, and vitamins. Through a feedback mechanism, the circulating T$_4$ level influences the release of TSH as well as thyrotropin-releasing hormone (TRH) from the hypothalamus. The FT$_4$ level is measured in preference to total T$_4$ because its measurement is not affected by blood protein levels. FT$_4$ is usually ordered after an abnormal TSH test has been returned, or when clinical suspicion of thyroid disease remains when the TSH is normal. TSH and FT$_4$ together suggest the following diagnoses: • TSH high, FT$_4$ low: hypothyroidism • TSH high, FT$_4$ normal: subclinical hypothyroidism • TSH low, FT$_4$ high: hyperthyroidism • TSH low, FT$_4$ normal: subclinical hyperthyroidism • TSH low, FT$_4$ low: nonthyroidal illness
Relevance to psychiatry and behavioral science	Elevated FT$_4$ with low TSH indicates hyperthyroidism, which is characterized by sometimes dramatic psychiatric symptoms, including mood disorders, psychosis, and delirium. The geriatric syndrome of apathetic hyperthyroidism is described in the Hyperthyroidism entry in Chapter 2, "Diseases and Conditions." Low FT$_4$ with elevated TSH indicates hypothyroidism, which is associated with fatigue, depression, and memory impairment. Low FT$_4$ with low TSH commonly accompanies nonthyroidal illness in acutely ill patients. Normal FT$_4$ with abnormal TSH is consistent with subclinical thyroid disease, which may manifest as a fully developed or *formes frustes* syndrome of hyperthyroidism or hypothyroidism.
Preparation of patient	None needed
Indications	• Abnormal TSH result • Signs/symptoms of thyroid disease (even if TSH is normal)

Thyroid function testing: free thyroxine (free T_4; FT_4) *(continued)*

Reference range	The reference range depends on the specific method used for assay; consult lab reference values. For patients taking levothyroxine, the upper limit of normal is 5.0 ng/dL (64 pmol/L).
Critical value(s)	None
Increased levels	• Hyperthyroidism (Graves disease) • Treated hypothyroidism • *Drugs:* aspirin, carbamazepine, furosemide, heparin, phenytoin, propranolol, X-ray contrast agents, and valproate
Decreased levels	• Primary hypothyroidism • Secondary hypothyroidism (pituitary cause) • Tertiary hypothyroidism (hypothalamic cause) • Hypothyroidism treated with triiodothyronine (T_3) • Late pregnancy • *Drugs:* carbamazepine, corticosteroids, estrogen, lithium, methadone, oral contraceptives, phenobarbital, and phenytoin
Interfering factors	FT_4 levels fluctuate in pregnancy and in severe or chronic illness. Different reference ranges apply in pregnancy.
Cross-references	Hyperthyroidism Hypothyroidism Thyroid Function Testing: Thyroid-Stimulating Hormone (TSH)

Biondi B, Palmieri EA, Klain M, et al: Subclinical hyperthyroidism: clinical features and treatment options. Eur J Endocrinol 152(1):1–9, 2005

Col NF, Surks MI, Daniels GH: Subclinical thyroid disease: clinical applications. JAMA 291(2):239–243, 2004

Roberts CG, Ladenson PW: Hypothyroidism. Lancet 363(9411):793–803, 2004

Thyroid function testing: thyroid-stimulating hormone (TSH)	
Type of test	Blood
Explanation of test	TSH secreted by the anterior pituitary gland stimulates the thyroid gland to release stored triiodothyronine (T_3) and thyroxine (T_4), hormones responsible for the regulation of metabolism. TSH secretion is in turn regulated by thyrotropin-releasing hormone (TRH) from the hypothalamus, and by feedback inhibition from T_3 and T_4. In the past, a combination of thyroid tests (thyroid panel) was used to screen for and diagnose thyroid disease, but the thyroid panel has now largely been replaced by the newer third- and fourth-generation TSH assays ("sensitive" and "highly sensitive" assays, respectively). When pituitary hypothyroidism is suspected, TSH should be assayed along with free T_4 (FT_4). When a thyroid disorder is suspected, the third-generation TSH is considered the best initial screening test. If the assay is normal, no further testing is indicated. If the assay is not normal, FT_4 is checked. TSH and FT_4 together suggest the following diagnoses: <ul><li>TSH high, FT_4 low: hypothyroidism</li><li>TSH high, FT_4 normal: subclinical hypothyroidism*</li><li>TSH low, FT_4 high: hyperthyroidism**</li><li>TSH low, FT_4 normal: subclinical hyperthyroidism</li><li>TSH low, FT_4 low: nonthyroidal illness</li></ul> *If TSH is high and FT_4 is normal, thyroid antibodies are checked. **If TSH is low and FT_4 is high, thyroid-stimulating immunoglobulin, thyroid peroxidase antibody, and TSH receptor antibody are checked.

Thyroid function testing:
thyroid-stimulating hormone (TSH) *(continued)*

Relevance to psychiatry and behavioral science	Low TSH with elevated FT_4 indicates hyperthyroidism, which is characterized by sometimes dramatic psychiatric symptoms, including anxiety and mood disorders, psychosis, and delirium. The geriatric syndrome of apathetic hyperthyroidism is described in the Hyperthyroidism entry in Chapter 2, "Diseases and Conditions." Elevated TSH with low FT_4 indicates hypothyroidism, which is associated with fatigue, depression, and memory impairment. Low TSH with low FT_4 commonly accompanies nonthyroidal illness in acutely ill patients. Abnormal TSH with normal FT_4 is consistent with subclinical thyroid disease, which may manifest as a fully developed or *formes frustes* syndrome of hyperthyroidism or hypothyroidism. Numerous psychotropic drugs affect the TSH level without causing disease.
Preparation of patient	None needed
Indications	• Diagnosing hypothyroidism or hyperthyroidism in a symptomatic patient • Screening for thyroid disease in patients at risk, such as women over age 50 years, patients with newly diagnosed type 2 diabetes, pregnant women, postpartum women, and patients treated with lithium • Monitoring the efficacy of thyroid replacement therapy in a patient with hypothyroidism • Standard component of the workup for patients with depression, memory impairment, or dementia • Assisting in the workup of female infertility
Reference range	Adults 21–54 years: 0.4–4.2 µU/mL (0.4–4.2 mU/L) Adults 55–87 years: 0.5–8.9 µU/mL (0.5–8.9 mU/L) Borderline hyperthyroidism: 0.1–0.29 µU/mL Probable hyperthyroidism: <0.1 µU/mL Borderline hypothyroidism: 5.1–7.0 µU/mL Probable hypothyroidism: >7.0 µU/mL Target level for T_4 replacement therapy: 0.5–3.5 µU/mL *Note:* With treatment for hypothyroid or hyperthyroid states, the TSH may remain abnormal for up to 6 weeks after a euthyroid state has been attained.
Critical value(s)	TSH<0.1 µU/mL indicates primary hyperthyroidism or exogenous thyrotoxicosis, with risk of atrial fibrillation (a major risk factor for stroke)

Thyroid function testing: thyroid-stimulating hormone (TSH) *(continued)*	
Increased levels	<ul><li>Primary hypothyroidism (up to 100 times normal)</li><li>TSH-producing tumor (e.g., breast or lung)</li><li>Hashimoto thyroiditis</li><li>Recovery phase of subacute thyroiditis or nonthyroidal illness</li><li>Insufficient thyroid replacement or thyroid hormone resistance in treated hypothyroid patients</li><li>*Drugs:* aripiprazole, atenolol, carbamazepine, chlorpromazine, estrogen, ferrous sulfate, haloperidol, iodine-containing drugs or foods, lithium, lovastatin, metoclopramide, morphine, phenothiazines, phenytoin, prednisone, propranolol, sumatriptan, and valproate, among other drugs</li></ul>
Decreased levels	<ul><li>Primary hyperthyroidism</li><li>Secondary hypothyroidism (pituitary disease)</li><li>Tertiary hypothyroidism (hypothalamic disease)</li><li>Subclinical hyperthyroidism (e.g., toxic multinodular goiter, treated Graves disease)</li><li>Euthyroid sick syndrome</li><li>Overreplacement of thyroid hormone in treated hypothyroid patients</li><li>*Drugs:* aspirin, carbamazepine, corticosteroids, hydrocortisone, or interferon-$\alpha 2$, among other drugs</li></ul>
Interfering factors	Increased TSH levels may be found in the elderly (for patients over 80 years, upper limit of normal is 10 μU/mL) and in amphetamine abusers. Decreased TSH levels may be found in conditions of extreme stress, in acute illness, and during the first trimester of pregnancy.
Cross-references	Hyperthyroidism Hypothyroidism Thyroid Function Testing: Free Thyroxine (Free T_4; FT_4)

Col NF, Surks MI, Daniels GH: Subclinical thyroid disease: clinical applications. JAMA 291(2):239–243, 2004

Roberts CG, Ladenson PW: Hypothyroidism. Lancet 363(9411):793–803, 2004

Spaulding SW, Lippes H: Hyperthyroidism. Causes, clinical features, and diagnosis. Med Clin North Am 69:937–951, 1985

Triglycerides

Type of test	Blood
Explanation of test	Most dietary fat intake is in the form of triglycerides, which serve as a major energy source for the body. At any given time, most triglyceride is stored in adipose tissue as glycerol, fatty acids, and monoglycerides. A smaller amount is in circulation, and this is what is measured in the assay. After a meal, triglyceride levels can increase dramatically as the body converts dietary energy into adipose tissue. Between meals, adipose tissue is reconverted to triglycerides for needed energy.
	High triglyceride levels are associated with heightened risk of cardiovascular disease and events such as heart attack and stroke. Certain medical and lifestyle factors are in turn associated with elevated triglyceride levels, including diabetes, kidney disease, lack of exercise, smoking, being overweight, and drinking too much alcohol.
	When triglycerides are measured, cholesterol is measured as well, as both represent risk factors for atherosclerotic disease, and the two can vary independently.
Relevance to psychiatry and behavioral science	Triglyceride levels may be elevated in alcoholism, anorexia nervosa, and stroke. In addition, psychotropic drugs such as mirtazapine, risperidone, and beta-blockers are associated with triglyceride elevations. Before such drugs are initiated, a fasting lipid profile should be obtained. High triglyceride levels also increase the patient's risk of pancreatitis.
Preparation of patient	The patient should fast overnight and should abstain from alcohol for 24 hours before the test.
Indications	• A component of the lipid panel, obtained every 5 years in healthy adults
	• Assessing risk of cardiovascular disease
	• Patients being considered for lipid-lowering treatment
	• Evaluating suspected atherosclerosis
	• Monitoring the effect of lipid-lowering treatment
	• Assessing the body's ability to metabolize fat
	• Baseline measurement in high-risk children (with a family history of diabetes, obesity, or hypertension) between 2 and 10 years of age
	• Before starting a drug known to increase triglycerides

Triglycerides *(continued)*	
Reference range	Normal: <150 mg/dL (<1.70 mmol/L)
	Borderline high: 150–199 mg/dL (1.70–2.25 mmol/L)
	High: 200–499 mg/dL (2.26–5.64 mmol/L)
	Very high: ≥500 mg/dL (≥5.65 mmol/L)
	Note: These norms are for *fasting* samples.
Critical value(s)	A level of >500 mg/dL (>5.6 mmol/L) represents an increased risk of pancreatitis.
	A level of >5,000 mg/dL (>56.5 mmol/L) is associated with eruptive xanthoma, arcus cornealis, enlarged liver and spleen, and lipemia retinalis.
Increased levels	• Hyperlipoproteinemia (types I, II-b, III, IV, and V)
	• Alcoholism
	• Liver disease
	• Kidney disease, nephrotic syndrome
	• Hypothyroidism
	• Poorly controlled diabetes
	• Pancreatitis
	• Glycogen storage disease
	• Myocardial infarction
	• Gout
	• Werner syndrome
	• Down syndrome
	• Anorexia nervosa
	• *Drugs:* beta-blockers, corticosteroids, estrogens, furosemide, hydrochlorothiazide, interferon-α2a, isotretinoin, mirtazapine, oral contraceptives, protease inhibitors, risperidone, and warfarin
Decreased levels	• Abetalipoproteinemia (congenital)
	• Malnutrition
	• Malabsorption
	• Hyperthyroidism
	• Hyperparathyroidism
	• Stroke

Triglycerides *(continued)*	
Decreased levels *(continued)*	• Chronic obstructive pulmonary disease • *Drugs:* angiotensin-converting enzyme (ACE) inhibitors, some cholesterol-lowering drugs, hydroxychloroquine, indomethacin, insulin, levodopa, niacin, and psyllium
Interfering factors	Food intake drastically increases triglyceride levels within hours of a meal. Alcohol increases triglyceride levels. Fasting levels may vary from day to day. A transient decrease occurs after strenuous exercise. Levels increase in pregnancy. Poorly controlled blood sugar in patients with diabetes can drive triglyceride levels up. Levels increase with acute illnesses such as colds or influenza.
Cross-references	Lipid Panel Metabolic Syndrome

Brunzell JD: Clinical practice. Hypertriglyceridemia. N Engl J Med 357(10):1009–1017, 2007
Yuan G, Al-Shali KZ, Hegele RA: Hypertriglyceridemia: its etiology, effects and treatment. CMAJ 176(8):1113–1120, 2007

Tuberculosis (TB) testing

Type of test	• Skin test (Mantoux, also known as purified protein derivative [PPD]) • Blood test (interferon-γ [IFN-γ] release assays) • Sputum smear/culture • Chest X-ray • Cerebrospinal fluid and/or other body fluid or tissue samples, as indicated (e.g., biopsy tissue, urine, joint aspirate)
Explanation of test	Tests used to detect TB infection include the TB skin test (Mantoux test) and the newer TB blood tests, which measure IFN-γ release in response to the presence of the TB bacillus. These latter tests, known by trade names such as QuantiFERON-TB Gold and T-SPOT.TB, can be used in the same way as the TB skin test. These tests are used for patients who have been vaccinated with BCG (bacille Calmette-Guerin), in whom the skin test may be positive because of the vaccine. When the skin test or one of the blood tests is positive, a workup for TB disease is done, including medical history, physical exam, chest X ray, and sputum sampling for acid-fast bacilli (AFB). Other body fluids and tissues are sampled as indicated. When sputum is collected, a standard practice is to obtain three morning samples on consecutive days. Each sample is viewed immediately as a smear; if AFB are present on any smear, then a mycobacterial infection is likely. The sample is cultured to identify the mycobacterium, and sensitivity to various drugs is determined. Positive identification of a species may take days to weeks, and negative results of no mycobacterial growth may take up to 8 weeks. In the patient treated for TB, AFB cultures can be used to monitor the effectiveness of treatment and determine when the patient's disease is no longer communicable.
Relevance to psychiatry and behavioral science	TB is a considerable public health risk for certain populations, including the homeless and those in nursing homes or correctional facilities. Elderly, very young, and immunocompromised patients are at particular risk. The index of suspicion for TB should be high in all psychiatric settings.
Preparation of patient	None needed

Indications	• Exposure to a person with active TB disease
	
	• HIV-positive or otherwise immunocompromised patient
	
	• Symptoms of active TB disease:
	  • Persistent cough
	  • Sputum or phlegm (may be blood-tinged)
	  • Unexplained weight loss
	  • Night sweats

Tuberculosis (TB) testing *(continued)*

Indications *(continued)*	• Recent immigration from a country where TB is endemic • Residence in a long-term care facility • Homelessness • Prisoner status • Intravenous drug use

Reference range	<10-mm area of induration on TB skin testing
	
	QuantiFERON-TB Gold:
	
	    Negative: <0.35 IU/mL IFN-γ
	
	    Positive: >0.35 IU/mL IFN-γ
	
	T-SPOT.TB: See report form.
	
	Sputum samples negative for AFB
	
	Chest X ray negative for TB
	
	Other tissue/fluid samples negative for AFB

Critical value(s)	None
Positive test	• *TB infection* is indicated by a positive skin test or blood test(s). • *TB disease* is indicated by a positive chest X ray or the presence of AFB in sputum or other tissue.
Negative test	When an AFB culture is negative in a patient suspected of having TB, either the patient does not have mycobacterial infection, the sampling did not successfully capture the bacilli, or the organism is present in some other body tissue. A negative culture several weeks after treatment indicates a positive response to treatment; in this case, the patient's infection is no longer communicable.
Interfering factors	Several conditions decrease responsiveness to the TB skin test and the QuantiFERON-TB Gold test: diabetes, silicosis, chronic renal failure, leukemia, and lymphoma. Treatment with immunosuppressive drugs also decreases responsiveness to the TB skin test.
Cross-reference	Tuberculosis (TB)

Franken WP, Timmermans JF, Prins C, et al: Comparison of Mantoux and QuantiFERON TB Gold tests for diagnosis of latent tuberculosis infection in Army personnel. Clin Vaccine Immunol 14(4):477–480, 2007

Park SY, Jeon K, Um SW, et al: Clinical utility of the QuantiFERON-TB Gold In-Tube test for the diagnosis of active pulmonary tuberculosis. Scand J Infect Dis 41(11–12):818–822, 2009

Piana F, Ruffo Codecasa L, Baldan R, et al: Use of T-SPOT.TB in latent tuberculosis infection diagnosis in general and immunosuppressed populations. New Microbiol 30(3):286–290, 2007

Uric acid	
Type of test	Blood
Explanation of test	Uric acid formed in the process of purine metabolism is transported in the blood from the liver to the kidneys, where most is excreted. The blood level can be elevated because of overproduction (e.g., gout or leukemia) or underexcretion (e.g., renal failure). Elevated uric acid is a risk factor for the development of hypertension, may have a role in the development of the metabolic syndrome, can cause renal disease even in the absence of urate crystal deposition, and is strongly associated with cerebrovascular disease, stroke, vascular dementia, and cardiovascular disease.
Relevance to psychiatry and behavioral science	Uric acid may be elevated in patients with alcoholism. High levels are strongly associated with hypertension, cardiovascular and cerebrovascular disease, stroke, and vascular dementia. High levels may have a role in the development of the metabolic syndrome. In addition, high levels predict poor outcome after stroke, including further events.
Preparation of patient	Ideally, the patient should fast for 8 hours before the test.
Indications	• Suspected gout • Monitoring effects of cytotoxic therapy • Evaluating renal failure
Reference range	Adult males: 4.4–7.6 mg/dL (262–452 µmol/L) Adult females: 2.3–6.6 mg/dL (137–393 µmol/L) Higher upper limits in adults ≥60 years Children <12 years: 2.0–5.5 mg/dL (119–327 µmol/L)
Critical value(s)	>12 mg/dL (>714 µmol/L)
Increased levels	• Gout • Leukemia, lymphoma, multiple myeloma • Hemolytic anemia, sickle cell anemia • Polycythemia vera • Psoriasis • Cytotoxic therapy • Starvation, anorexia nervosa, severe dieting • Renal failure • Alcoholism or alcohol consumption • Liver disease

Uric acid *(continued)*	
Increased levels *(continued)*	• Hyperlipidemia, obesity, metabolic syndrome • Metabolic acidosis, diabetic ketoacidosis • Pernicious anemia • Kidney stones • Lead poisoning • Purine-rich diet (enriched with red meat, seafood) • *Drugs:* diuretics, beta-blockers, aspirin
Decreased levels	• Fanconi syndrome • Wilson disease • Syndrome of inappropriate antidiuretic hormone secretion (SIADH) • Low purine diet • Certain malignancies (e.g., Hodgkin's disease, bronchogenic carcinoma) • Xanthinuria
Interfering factors	High levels of stress and strenuous exercise cause increased uric acid levels.
Cross-reference	Alcohol Use Disorder (Alcoholism)

Urinalysis (UA)	
Type of test	Urine
Explanation of test	A complete UA reports the following characteristics of urine: color, appearance, specific gravity, pH, glucose, ketones, blood, protein, bilirubin, urobilinogen, nitrite, leukocyte esterase, and findings from microscopic exam. The microscopic exam includes red blood cells (RBCs), white blood cells (WBCs), casts, crystals, and epithelial cells.
	Physical characteristics of the specimen are first noted, then chemical tests are performed, and finally the specimen is examined microscopically. The first two steps can be done using a dipstick and automated methods, which makes this test quick and cheap. The UA is often a standard component of the hospital admission workup or presurgical evaluation. Although its primary utility is in the diagnosis of urinary tract infection (UTI), information can be obtained from the UA about liver and kidney function as well as other health conditions.
Relevance to psychiatry and behavioral science	UA is a routine component of the workup for mental status changes, particularly in elderly patients in nursing homes or hospital settings. UTI can be associated with delirium, even in the absence of sepsis.
Preparation of patient	The patient's first morning specimen is preferred; 10 mL of urine constitutes a sufficient sample. The patient should be instructed to void directly into a clean, dry container. It is no longer recommended that the patient use antibacterial wipes to clean the perineum before voiding. Medications must be noted on the UA request form to aid in crystal identification by the laboratory. If a random sample is used, it should be collected at least 4 hours after the last voiding to ensure adequate contact time between bacteria and nitrates.
Indications	• Often a routine part of workup for hospital admission or preoperative surgical evaluation
	• Symptoms of UTI (irritation, burning, pain, change in frequency, or change in appearance of urine)
	• Recurrent UTI
	• Suspected pyelonephritis
	• Failed antibiotic treatment for UTI
	• Catheterized patients with fever, rigors, vomiting, confusion, or costovertebral angle tenderness
	• Screening for asymptomatic bacteriuria in pregnancy (at first antenatal visit)

Urinalysis (UA) *(continued)*	
Indications *(continued)*	• In children: unexplained fever, hypertension, urinary symptoms, hematuria, abdominal pain, loin pain, vomiting, or suspected sexual abuse • In elderly patients: fever, dysuria, incontinence (or increased frequency or urgency)
Reference range	Color: pale yellow to amber Appearance: clear to slightly hazy Specific gravity: 1.002–1.035 pH: 4.5–8.0 Glucose: negative Ketones: negative Blood: negative Protein: negative Bilirubin: negative Urobilinogen: negative (0–0.02 mg/dL or 0–0.34 µmol/L) Nitrite for bacteria: negative Leukocyte esterase: negative Casts: negative or an occasional hyaline RBCs: negative or rare Crystals: negative (none) WBCs: negative or rare Epithelial cells: few
Critical value(s)	A positive test for blood requires confirmation on a second sample and further investigation. Persistent or significant hematuria is defined as follows: • >3 RBCs/hpf on three urinalyses, or • >100 RBCs/hpf on a single UA, or • Gross hematuria. RBC casts indicate glomerular injury or, less commonly, severe tubular damage, among other conditions (e.g., congestive heart failure, malignant hypertension, lupus nephritis, acute bacterial endocarditis). Urine protein >150 mg/24 hours defines proteinuria (1+ to 4+). >2 g/24 hours in adults usually indicates glomerular etiology.

Urinalysis (UA) *(continued)*

Critical value(s) *(continued)*	>3.5 g/24 hours is consistent with nephrotic syndrome (with hypoalbuminemia, edema, and hyperlipidemia).
	Urine glucose>1,000 mg/dL (4+) indicates a need to check blood glucose immediately and begin prompt treatment.
	Presence of urinary ketones in a child less than 2 years of age requires immediate attention.
	Microalbuminuria: 30–300 mg/day (or increased microalbumin/creatinine ratio of 30–350 mg/g). Two of three urine samples taken over several months should have elevated microalbumin to confirm the finding of microalbuminuria.
	Specific gravity>1.035 indicates a contaminated specimen, high glucose concentration, or recent use of radiopaque dyes or intravenous low-molecular-weight dextran. Specific gravity≤1.022 after a 12-hour fast (no food or water) indicates impaired renal concentrating ability.
	>30 WBCs/hpf indicates the presence of an acute bacterial infection in the genitourinary system. The presence of WBC casts requires further investigation to rule out pyelonephritis, which may otherwise be asymptomatic.
Interfering factors	Improper specimen handling invalidates results. The urine must be examined within 1 hour of collection or refrigerated immediately and examined within 24 hours. If the first morning specimen is not used, inadequate contact time can yield a false-negative nitrite test. With clean-catch urine, feces, vaginal discharge, or menstrual blood can contaminate the specimen.
Cross-references	None

Misdraji J, Nguyen PL: Urinalysis. When—and when not—to order. Postgrad Med 100(1):173–176, 181–182, 185–188 passim, 1996

Simerville JA, Maxted WC, Pahira JJ: Urinalysis: a comprehensive review. Am Fam Physician 71(6):1153–1162, 2005

Valproate level	
Type of test	Blood
Explanation of test	Valproate is an antiepileptic drug indicated for generalized tonic-clonic, partial complex, and petit mal seizures. It is also used for bipolar disorder, mood instability in the context of dementia, traumatic brain injury, myoclonus, and many other neuropsychiatric disorders. The free valproate level should be checked in preference to the routine valproate level when there is any concern about altered or unpredictable protein-binding capacity.
Relevance to psychiatry and behavioral science	Reference ranges reported for valproate relate to seizure rather than behavioral indications. As a general rule, levels correlate poorly with mood and behavioral control. The reason that levels are checked in psychiatric practice is to monitor compliance (to exclude very low or zero levels) or toxicity (to exclude levels that are orders of magnitude above the upper limit of normal for seizure). Other "safety labs" are monitored, however, when valproate is used, as discussed in the Valproate entry in Chapter 3, "Psychotropic Medications."
Preparation of patient	The patient should be instructed to hold the dose of valproate until the blood level is drawn, just before the dose is due.
Indications	• Overdose • Signs/symptoms of valproate toxicity • Concern regarding noncompliance
Reference range	Total valproate 50–125 µg/mL Free valproate 5–25 µg/mL % Free valproate 5%–18% (calculated)
Critical value(s)	Total valproate >150 µg/mL Free valproate ≥30 µg/mL
Increased levels	• Overdose • Hepatic failure • *Drugs:* fluoxetine
Decreased levels	• Noncompliance • *Drugs:* carbamazepine
Interfering factors	None
Cross-references	Manic Episode Valproate

Vitamin B$_{12}$

Type of test	Blood
Explanation of test	Vitamin B$_{12}$ is needed at adequate levels for proper digestion and absorption of food, protein synthesis, fat and carbohydrate metabolism, formation of iron, production of acetylcholine, maintenance of nerve cells, and fertility. Vitamin B$_{12}$ deficiency due to inadequate intake is rare in developed countries. Deficiency usually is due to malabsorption, which is common in elderly patients and also can occur with cystic fibrosis, pernicious anemia, reduced gastric acid production, excessive use of antacids or chronic use of histamine$_2$ blockers or proton pump inhibitors, after gastric bypass surgery, and with other gastrointestinal conditions (e.g., tapeworm). Increased loss of B$_{12}$ may be seen in alcoholism and in liver and kidney disease. A deficiency may be associated with a megaloblastic anemia, where fewer and larger red blood cells are produced. The syndrome of subacute combined degeneration of the spinal cord due to B$_{12}$ deficiency is discussed in the Vitamin B$_{12}$ Deficiency entry in Chapter 2, "Diseases and Conditions."
Relevance to psychiatry and behavioral science	Vitamin B$_{12}$ deficiency is associated with a variety of symptoms of interest to psychiatrists and other behavioral health practitioners, including confusion, delirium, psychosis, somnolence, irritability, depression, mania, apathy, personality change, delusions, cognitive impairment (particularly involving memory), and nonspecific symptoms of dizziness, weakness, and fatigue. Patients with vague neurological symptoms such as clumsiness, unsteadiness, tinnitus, speech impairment, or visual changes are sometimes misdiagnosed with somatoform disorders.
Preparation of patient	The patient should fast overnight before the test and on the day of testing should hold heparin and avoid vitamin C, fluoride, and alcohol.
Indications	• A standard component of the workup for dementia or memory impairment • Identifying cause of delirium • Evaluating mental status changes in an elderly patient • Identifying cause of peripheral neuropathy • Presence of symptoms of subacute combined degeneration (weakness, sensory abnormalities) • Workup for macrocytic anemia* • Workup for macrocytosis (mean corpuscular volume >110 fL)* • Evaluating nutritional status • Monitoring effectiveness of treatment for vitamin B$_{12}$ deficiency *If the patient also has macrocytosis or anemia, check folate.

Vitamin B$_{12}$ *(continued)*	
Reference range	250–1,000 pg/mL (180–740 pmol/L)
Critical value(s)	For geriatric patients or adult patients with neurological or psychiatric symptoms listed in the "Relevance" section above, many clinicians will prescribe vitamin B$_{12}$ supplementation when levels are <400 pg/mL.
Increased levels	• Supplementation • Leukemia • Liver dysfunction High B$_{12}$ levels have not been associated with toxicity and are of uncertain significance.
Decreased levels	• Inadequate intake (e.g., vegetarian diet) • Poor absorption • Increased excretion • *Drugs:* anticonvulsants, ascorbic acid, cholestyramine, chlorpromazine, colchicine, levodopa, metformin, neomycin, octreotide, oral contraceptives, ranitidine, or rifampin
Interfering factors	None
Cross-references	Folate Folate Deficiency Vitamin B$_{12}$ Deficiency

Hvas AM, Nexo E: Diagnosis and treatment of vitamin B$_{12}$ deficiency—an update. Haematologica 91(11):1506–1512, 2006

Lerner V, Kanevsky M, Dwolatzky T, et al: Vitamin B$_{12}$ and folate serum levels in newly admitted psychiatric patients. Clin Nutr 25(1):60–67, 2006

Vitamin D	
Type of test	Blood
Explanation of test	Vitamin D is a fat-soluble vitamin ingested in foods and supplements and synthesized in the skin on exposure to sunlight. It becomes biologically active through hydroxylation in the liver and kidneys. Vitamin D works with other hormones to regulate calcium balance (absorption from the gastrointestinal tract and resorption from bone) and also to regulate phosphorus and magnesium absorption. Adequate levels of vitamin D are needed at all ages for bone growth and health. In older age, women are particularly prone to develop deficiency, especially those with dark skin, those who lack sunlight exposure, and those with malabsorption. The 25-OH vitamin D level by chemiluminescence is the recommended assay.
Relevance to psychiatry and behavioral science	Vitamin D deficiency is associated with failure to thrive in children and weakness in geriatric patients. An estimated one-third of older adults are deficient. Deficiency is particularly common among women in nursing home populations. An association of deficiency with Alzheimer's disease has been noted. Symptoms of deficiency are for the most part nonpsychiatric, but involve bones, heart, and the risk of developing certain cancers and autoimmune diseases.
Preparation of patient	The patient should fast overnight before the test.
Indications	• Detecting vitamin D deficiency in patients at risk • Confirming deficiency in patients with evidence of bone disease, bone or muscle weakness, or abnormal calcium, phosphorus, and/or parathyroid hormone levels • Monitoring effectiveness of vitamin D replacement
Reference range	Depends on testing method: *High-performance liquid chromatography (HPLC), competitive protein binding (CPB), or radioimmunoassay (RIA)* 14–60 ng/mL (35–150 nmol/L) *Liquid chromatography–tandem mass spectrometry (LC-MS/MS)* Severe deficiency: <10 ng/mL (<25 nmol/L) Mild-moderate deficiency: 10–24 ng/mL (25–60 nmol/L) Optimal level: 25–80 ng/mL (61–200 nmol/L)

Vitamin D *(continued)*

Critical value(s)	Toxicity is possible with 25-OH vitamin D levels >150 ng/mL (>375 nmol/L). These levels can be associated with tissue calcification (e.g., kidneys, vasculature), vomiting, constipation, anorexia, nausea, severe electrolyte derangement, and retarded growth and mental retardation (intellectual disability) in infants and children.
Increased levels	• Excessive supplementation
Decreased levels	• Inadequate vitamin D intake • Malabsorption of vitamin D (a fat-soluble vitamin) • Inadequate sunlight exposure • *Drugs:* anticonvulsants (carbamazepine, phenytoin, primidone, phenobarbital), aluminum hydroxide, cholestyramine, glucocorticoids, isoniazid (INH), rifampin, or mineral oil
Interfering factors	None
Cross-references	None

Zerwekh JE: Blood biomarkers of vitamin D status. Am J Clin Nutr 87(4):1087S–1091S, 2008

White blood cell count (WBC)

Type of test	Blood
Explanation of test	White blood cells are immune system cells that help fight infection and foreign material introduced into the body. These cells are capable of encapsulating and destroying organisms as well as producing and transporting antibodies. When these processes occur, the WBC increases, with the degree of elevation corresponding to the severity of infection. There are five types of WBCs—basophils, eosinophils, lymphocytes, monocytes, and neutrophils—present in fairly stable proportions. Usually, when the WBC is elevated, only one of the five types is actually increased in number. If all cell types are increased in number, it is most likely that hemoconcentration has occurred.
Relevance to psychiatry and behavioral science	Delirium is associated with conditions involving both elevated and decreased WBC levels. Lithium often causes leukocytosis. Clozapine and other psychotropic drugs may cause leukopenia or agranulocytosis. In general, patients with persistent leukopenia require special care, including protection from fresh fruits and vegetables, plants and flowers, intramuscular injections, rectal thermometers or suppositories, tooth flossing, razor blades, and aspirin and nonsteroidal anti-inflammatory drugs.
Preparation of patient	Fasting is not required. Any physiological stress should be avoided just prior to the test.
Indications	• A routine component of the complete blood count • May be ordered as an individual test (with neutrophil count) for clozapine monitoring
Reference range	Children 6–18 years: $4.8–10.8 \times 10^3$ cells/mm^3 African American adults: $3.2–10.0 \times 10^3$ cells/mm^3 Adults other than African Americans: $4.5–10.5 \times 10^3$ cells/mm^3
Critical value(s)	$<2.0 \times 10^3$ cells/mm^3 ($<0.5 \times 10^3$ cells/mm^3 extremely dangerous, often fatal) $>30.0 \times 10^3$ cells/mm^3

White blood cell count (WBC) *(continued)*	
Increased levels	Leukocytosis (WBC count $>11.0 \times 10^3$ cells/mm^3) occurs in the following conditions: acute infection, leukemia, myelo-proliferative disorders, tissue trauma, surgery, cancer (especially bronchogenic carcinoma), uremia, coma, eclampsia, thyrotoxicosis, ingestion of toxins, use of certain medications (lithium, corticosteroids, epinephrine, colony-stimulating factors, quinine), neuroleptic malignant syndrome, acute hemolysis, acute hemorrhage, postsplenectomy, poly-cythemia vera, tissue necrosis, seizure, nausea and vomiting, physiological leukocytosis (e.g., from stress, exercise, pain, heat/cold), and sunlight exposure.
Decreased levels	Leukopenia (WBC count $<4.0 \times 10^3$ cells/mm^3) occurs in the following conditions: viral infections, certain bacterial infections, overwhelming bacterial infections, hypersplenism, primary bone marrow disorders (including leukemia, aplastic anemia, and pernicious anemia), and bone marrow depression by heavy metal intoxication, radiation, or drugs.
Interfering factors	A diurnal rhythm is seen, with early-morning trough WBC levels and late-afternoon peaks. WBC values are also influenced by age, gender, exercise, medications, pregnancy, pain, temperature, altitude, and anesthesia. Any stress that increases endogenous epinephrine levels also increases the WBC level.
Cross-reference	Complete Blood Count (CBC)

Wilson disease screening panel

Type of test	Blood
Explanation of test	Wilson disease is an autosomal recessive inherited disorder of copper metabolism in which circulating free copper levels are elevated. Excess copper is deposited in the brain, eyes, liver, and kidneys, giving rise to characteristic signs and symptoms. The screening panel includes serum ceruloplasmin, serum copper, and the calculated free serum copper. Other tests that may be useful include 24-hour urine copper, hepatic copper, and genetic testing for the *ATP7B* mutation. In Wilson disease, serum ceruloplasmin is usually low, and the free copper level is usually high (>25 µg/dL).
Relevance to psychiatry and behavioral science	Neuropsychiatric symptoms of Wilson disease are often prominent and may precede other disease manifestations. Psychosis, depression, and behavioral problems may be seen. Abnormal movements and motor system abnormalities include dystonia, tremor, incoordination, hypokinetic speech, dysphagia, and bulbar and pseudobulbar palsies.
Preparation of patient	None needed
Indications	• Clinical suspicion of Wilson disease • Family history of Wilson disease • Early onset of hepatitis or cirrhosis • Neuropsychiatric symptoms consistent with Wilson disease

Reference range	*Ceruloplasmin*
	
	  18–45 mg/dL (240–560 mg/L)
	
	Serum copper
	
	  Children: 30–150 µg/dL (4.71–23.5 µmol/L)
	
	  Adult males: 70–140 µg/dL (11.0–22.0 µmol/L)
	
	  Adult females: 80–155 µg/dL (12.6–24.3 µmol/L)
	
	  Levels are higher in patients over age 60 years.
	
	Serum free copper:
	
	Calculated as the difference between serum copper concentration (in µg/dL) and 3× ceruloplasmin concentration (in mg/dL). Normal free copper value is <15 µg/dL.

Critical values	Serum free copper >25 µg/dL is consistent with Wilson disease.

Wilson disease screening panel *(continued)*

Positive test	Decreased ceruloplasmin and increased free copper (also increased urine copper and presence of Kayser-Fleischer rings) confirm the diagnosis of Wilson disease. In these cases, liver biopsy can be used to quantitate copper, although this is not required for the diagnosis. Treatment should be initiated. Genetic tests should be considered for the patient and family members. If the results are equivocal, liver biopsy with copper quantitation can be used to confirm the diagnosis. If the liver copper level is ≥250 µg/g and histology is consistent with Wilson disease, the diagnosis is confirmed. If the copper level is <250 µg/g and histology is not consistent with Wilson disease, an alternate diagnosis should be considered and/or the patient should be reevaluated in 3–6 months.
Negative test	Normal ceruloplasmin and free copper levels (also normal urine copper level and normal liver function tests) in a patient ≥15 years of age indicates an alternate diagnosis. A patient under 15 years should be reevaluated in 3–6 months.
Interfering factors	Elevated copper levels from tubes not certified metal-free might be due to contamination. Elevated levels should be confirmed with a second specimen collected in a metal-free tube. In pregnancy, serum ceruloplasmin values gradually increase and may peak at levels up to three times normal. Ceruloplasmin is an acute-phase reactant and is increased in inflammation, infection, tissue injury, malignancy, and cardiovascular disease. Drugs associated with elevated ceruloplasmin levels include anticonvulsants, estrogens, methadone, and nicotine. Drugs associated with elevated copper levels include anticonvulsants and estrogens.
Cross-references	None

CHAPTER 2

Diseases and Conditions

Alcohol use disorder (alcoholism)

Clinical diagnosis	Based on clinical history and physical examination findings
Laboratory testing	Laboratory abnormalities that support the diagnosis of alcoholism that is suspected on clinical grounds include the following: • Elevated gamma-glutamyltransferase (GGT) (>47 U/L in men or >25 U/L in women) is consistent with four or more drinks daily for 4 weeks or more. It takes 2–3 weeks of abstinence to normalize the GGT level. • Elevated carbohydrate-deficient transferrin (CDT): ≥2.6% • Elevated ratio of aspartate transaminase (AST) to alanine transaminase (ALT) (AST : ALT > 2:1) • Elevated mean corpuscular volume (MCV) (>101 fL, although this is age- and gender-dependent) • Elevated uric acid level (≥7 mg/dL, although this is age- and gender-dependent) • Elevated total homocysteine level (>15 μmol/L) Recent drinking can be confirmed using breath analysis, saliva ethanol, urine ethanol, or blood alcohol level (BAL). Urine ethylglucuronide can also be measured; this metabolite of ethanol remains positive in urine for 2–3 days. GGT and/or CDT can also be useful. In males, GGT and CDT together provide a reliable indicator; in females, GGT alone has better predictive value. GGT and CDT begin to normalize within days of cessation of drinking, and they return to normal levels within 2 weeks. In the patient with known alcohol dependence or abuse, BAL may be useful in diagnosing intoxication or withdrawal (the latter when BAL is zero in the presence of relevant signs and symptoms). Common blood lab abnormalities in the patient with alcoholism include the following: • Hypomagnesemia • Hypophosphatemia • Hypoglycemia • Anemia • Thrombocytopenia • Hypoprothrombinemia In alcohol-related dementia, computed tomography (CT) or magnetic resonance imaging (MRI) may show generalized atrophy (both cortical and central atrophy, the latter evidenced by ventricular enlargement). Atrophy may decrease to some extent with abstinence.

Alcohol use disorder (alcoholism) *(continued)*

Laboratory testing *(continued)*	In cerebellar degeneration, CT or MRI may show atrophy of the cerebellar cortex, most often in the anterior and superior segments of the vermis. The radiologist should be alerted to clinical findings suggestive of cerebellar involvement.
	The clinical diagnosis of alcohol-related polyneuropathy can be confirmed by electromyography (EMG), with single-fiber study complementing conventional needle EMG.
	In acute alcoholic myopathy, AST and creatine kinase may be elevated in the presence of painful muscle weakness. Chronic alcohol-related myopathy, which is progressive with continued drinking, can be diagnosed by EMG or nerve conduction testing. Patients with recurrent seizures or who are "found down" may develop rhabdomyolysis with myoglobinuria and acute renal failure.

Brust JC: A 74-year-old man with memory loss and neuropathy who enjoys alcoholic beverages. JAMA 299(9):1046–1054, 2008

Rinck D, Frieling H, Freitag A, et al: Combinations of carbohydrate-deficient transferrin, mean corpuscular erythrocyte volume, gamma-glutamyltransferase, homocysteine and folate increase the significance of biological markers in alcohol dependent patients. Drug Alcohol Depend 89(1):60–65, 2007

Sillanaukee P: Laboratory markers of alcohol abuse. Alcohol Alcohol 31(6):613–616, 1996

Anorexia nervosa	
Clinical diagnosis	Restriction of energy intake relative to requirements, leading to a significantly low body weight. Intense fear of gaining weight or becoming fat or persistent behavior that interferes with weight gain, even though at a significantly low weight. Disturbance in the way in which one's body weight or shape is experienced, undue influence of body weight or shape on self-evaluation, or persistent lack of recognition of the seriousness of the current low body weight. Restricting or binge-eating/purging subtypes are specified.
Laboratory testing	For all patients with eating disorders: • Complete blood count with differential • Blood chemistries: electrolytes • Blood urea nitrogen (BUN), creatinine • Liver function tests (LFTs): aspartate transaminase (AST), alanine transaminase (ALT), alkaline phosphatase (ALP) • Thyroid-stimulating hormone: free T_4, T_3 if indicated • Erythrocyte sedimentation rate • Urinalysis Consider for malnourished and severely symptomatic patients: • Blood chemistries: calcium, magnesium, phosphorus (derangements) • Thiamine level (low) • LFTs (elevated AST, lactate dehydrogenase [LDH], ALP) • Electrocardiogram (may show bradycardia, prolonged QT interval, nonspecific ST-segment changes, U waves, and, in severe cases, dysrhythmias, including ventricular fibrillation and asystole) Consider for patients underweight more than 6 months: • Dual-energy X-ray absorptiometry (DEXA) scan for osteoporosis/osteopenia • Estradiol level • Testosterone level in males

Anorexia nervosa *(continued)*	
Laboratory testing *(continued)*	Nonroutine assessments: • Serum amylase level (may indicate persistent or recurrent vomiting) • Luteinizing hormone and follicle-stimulating hormone levels (for persistent amenorrhea at normal weight) • Brain magnetic resonance imaging or computed tomography (to detect ventricular enlargement correlated with degree of malnutrition) • Fecal occult blood testing (may be positive in individuals with purging behaviors)

American Psychiatric Association: Practice Guidelines for the Treatment of Psychiatric Disorders. Washington, DC, American Psychiatric Association, 2000b

Treasure J, Claudino AM, Zucker N: Eating disorders. Lancet 375(9714):583–593, 2010

Yager J, Andersen AE: Clinical practice: anorexia nervosa. N Engl J Med 353(14):1481–1488, 2005

Anxiety disorder (secondary): substance/medication-induced or due to another medical condition

Clinical diagnosis	Prominent anxiety symptoms or panic attacks are characteristic. Secondary anxiety may be chronic and unremitting, or it may be episodic. Causes of chronic secondary anxiety include chronic obstructive pulmonary disease, hyperthyroidism, hypocalcemia, congestive heart failure, traumatic brain injury, dementia, and stroke (especially left frontal). Drugs associated with chronic secondary anxiety include stimulants, yohimbine, and antidepressants in certain patients (especially if dose is excessive). Also associated is withdrawal from clonidine, anticholinergic drugs, alcohol, sedative-hypnotics, and nicotine.
	Causes of episodic secondary anxiety include Parkinson's disease (during "off" periods), angina (especially in women), asthma, paroxysmal atrial tachycardia, pheochromocytoma, hypoglycemia, substance abuse or withdrawal, simple partial seizures, pulmonary emboli, and mastocytosis. Drugs associated with episodic secondary anxiety include sympathomimetics, caffeine, cocaine, amphetamines, marijuana, and hallucinogens. Also associated is withdrawal from alcohol (which may occur at a particular time every day after the previous night's drinking).
Laboratory testing	The basic laboratory workup for secondary anxiety includes only a metabolic panel (basic metabolic panel or comprehensive metabolic panel) to check calcium and glucose levels, and thyroid-stimulating hormone (TSH).
	Depending on patient characteristics and history, other elements of the evaluation might include one or more of the following:
	• Electrocardiogram, Holter monitoring, cardiac stress testing, and/or echocardiogram
	• Chest X ray, pulmonary function tests, and/or arterial blood gases
	• Gamma-glutamyltransferase with or without carbohydrate-deficient transferrin (%CDT) for suspicion of covert drinking
	• Plasma free metanephrines
	• Urine porphyrin precursors (aminolevulinic acid and porphobilinogen)
	• Pulmonary computed tomography scan
	• Electroencephalogram

Attention-deficit/hyperactivity disorder (ADHD)	
Clinical diagnosis	ADHD is characterized by a pattern of inattention and/or hyperactivity-impulsivity that has persisted for at least 6 months, is inconsistent with developmental level, and impacts directly on social, academic, or occupational activities. *Inattention* is defined by the following symptoms, six of which must be present (five in those age 17 years or older): fails to give close attention to details, has difficulty sustaining attention, does not seem to listen, does not follow through, has difficulty organizing tasks, is reluctant to engage in tasks requiring sustained mental effort, loses objects needed for tasks or activities, is easily distracted, is forgetful in daily activities. *Hyperactivity/impulsivity* is defined by the following symptoms, six of which must be present (five in those age 17 years or older): often fidgets, leaves seat when remaining seated is expected, runs about or climbs when it is inappropriate (may be limited to feeling restless in older patients), is unable to engage in leisure activities quietly, is often "on the go," talks excessively, blurts out answers before questions are complete (completes people's sentences), has difficulty waiting his or her turn, interrupts or intrudes on others. Several symptoms were present by age 12, and symptoms are apparent in two or more settings. Symptoms interfere with social, academic, or occupational functioning. Subtype is specified: combined, predominantly inattentive, or predominantly hyperactive/impulsive.
Laboratory testing	Tests may be used to exclude certain conditions that can mimic ADHD symptoms: • Drug use—urine drug screen (Note: will not detect inhalant use) • Traumatic brain injury—magnetic resonance imaging (MRI) • Epilepsy—electroencephalogram (EEG) and/or EEG monitoring • Hydrocephalus—computed tomography (CT) or MRI • Brain aneurysm or arteriovenous malformation—CT or MRI • Stroke—CT or MRI • HIV testing • Thyroid disease—thyroid-stimulating hormone • Lead poisoning—blood lead level • Vision and hearing testing • Pediatric autoimmune neuropsychiatric disorders associated with streptococcal infections (PANDAS)—antistreptolysin-O titer and other tests

American Psychiatric Association: Diagnostic and Statistical Manual of Mental Disorders, 5th Edition. Arlington, VA, American Psychiatric Association, 2013.

Autism spectrum disorder (ASD)	
Clinical diagnosis	ASD is characterized by the following: • Clinically significant, persistent *deficits in social communication and interactions*, as manifested by all of the following: deficits in social-emotional reciprocity, deficits in nonverbal and verbal communication used for social interaction, and deficits in developing, maintaining, and understanding relationships • *Restricted, repetitive patterns of behavior, interests, or activities*, as manifested by at least two of the following: stereotyped or repetitive motor movements, use of objects, or speech; insistence on sameness, inflexible adherence to routines, or ritualized patterns of verbal or nonverbal behavior; highly restricted, fixated interests that are abnormal in intensity or focus; hyper- or hyporeactivity to sensory input or unusual interest in sensory aspects of the environment Symptoms of ASD must be present in the early developmental period, but they may not become fully manifest until social demands exceed limited capacities or may be masked by learned strategies in later life.
Laboratory testing	Lintas and Persico (2009) suggested guidelines for genetic counseling and testing for ASD, with highlights as follows: • If a couple has an autistic child without clear etiology (e.g., in the absence of fragile X or other cause), the probability that a second child will also be autistic is approximately 5%–6%. • A karyotype and fragile X testing should be requested for all patients with ASD. • Prenatal genetic testing typically raises unrealistic expectations in parents of children with ASD because most genetic or genomic anomalies responsible for ASD are not detected using current prenatal screening methods. • In the presence of dysmorphic features and neurological symptoms, it is reasonable to suspect chromosomal rearrangements even if the karyotype appears normal. Depending on availability and cost, a bacterial artificial chromosome or oligonucleotide array–based comparative genomic hybridization analysis is strongly advised in these cases. Information about laboratories offering ASD genetic testing can be found at www.genetests.org.

American Psychiatric Association: Diagnostic and Statistical Manual of Mental Disorders, 5th Edition. Arlington, VA, American Psychiatric Association, 2013.

Buxbaum JD: Multiple rare variants in the etiology of autism spectrum disorders. Dialogues Clin Neurosci 11:35–43, 2009

Lintas C, Persico AM: Autistic phenotypes and genetic testing: state-of-the-art for the clinical geneticist. J Med Genet 46:1–8, 2009

Catatonia disorder due to another medical condition	
Clinical diagnosis	Catatonia is a syndrome that can occur in association with another mental disorder or another medical condition. The clinical picture is dominated by at least three of the following symptoms: • Stupor • Catalepsy • Waxy flexibility • Mutism • Negativism • Posturing • Mannerism • Stereotypy • Agitation • Grimacing • Echolalia • Echopraxia There is evidence from the history, physical examination, or laboratory findings that the disturbance is the direct pathophysiological consequence of another medical condition. It is not better accounted for by another mental disorder such as a manic episode, and does not occur exclusively during the course of a delirium. The disturbance causes clinically significant distress or impairment in social, occupational, or other important areas of functioning.
Laboratory testing	Laboratory workup is indicated to exclude a medical or substance-related cause of catatonia. Medical conditions associated with catatonia include nonconvulsive status epilepticus (NCSE), cancer, traumatic brain injury, encephalitis, cerebrovascular disease, and metabolic derangements such as hyponatremia, hypercalcemia, hepatic encephalopathy, and diabetic ketoacidosis. Medications known to cause catatonia include corticosteroids, immunosuppressants, and antipsychotics. Catatonic symptoms may be seen in neuroleptic malignant syndrome (NMS). Lab testing may include the following: • Complete blood count • Comprehensive metabolic panel • Creatine kinase (elevated in NMS) • Brain imaging (computed tomography or MRI) • Electroencephalogram if NCSE is suspected

American Psychiatric Association: Diagnostic and Statistical Manual of Mental Disorders, 5th Edition. Arlington, VA, American Psychiatric Association, 2013

Delirium	
Clinical diagnosis	The syndrome of delirium is characterized by the following: • A disturbance in attention and awareness • Develops over a short period of time (hours to days), represents a change from baseline, and fluctuates in severity • Involves an additional disturbance in cognitive functions such as memory, orientation, language, visuospatial ability, or perception Diseases underlying the syndrome of delirium include (but are not limited to) the following: infection (particularly sepsis, pneumonia, or urinary tract infection), metabolic derangement, electrolyte disturbance, dehydration, cardiac dysrhythmia, heart failure, stroke, myocardial infarction, traumatic brain injury, alcohol/sedative withdrawal, status epilepticus, and medication toxicity (e.g., with opioids or anticholinergics). Delirium also commonly occurs following major surgery, particularly heart surgery.
Laboratory testing	If the diagnosis of the syndrome of delirium is in doubt, an electroencephalogram (EEG) may be helpful in differentiating delirium from psychosis, catatonia, or dementia with behavioral disturbance. Most lab testing is performed to discover the medical cause(s) of delirium. For this purpose, the following tests usually are performed: • Comprehensive metabolic panel • Complete blood count with differential and platelets • Urinalysis (in women) In elderly patients and in nonelderly patients with cardiopulmonary symptoms, the following also are obtained: • Electrocardiogram • Chest X ray If this standard workup is unrevealing of a substantial cause of delirium, additional history should be obtained, and the following lab studies considered: • Erythrocyte sedimentation rate or C-reactive protein • Serum ammonia level • HIV testing • Antinuclear antibody test • Vitamin B_{12} and folate levels • Rapid plasma reagin • Urine toxicology • Blood alcohol level

Delirium *(continued)*	
Laboratory testing *(continued)*	• Medication levels • Brain magnetic resonance imaging (MRI) (or head computed tomography if MRI is contraindicated) • EEG if not done previously In the appropriate clinical setting, further consideration could be given to cerebrospinal fluid analysis, urine porphyrins, arterial blood gases, and blood cultures. Functional neuroimaging also is abnormal in delirium, showing global hypometabolism and reduction of cerebral blood flow that correlates with severity. These studies often are not captured in the delirious patient because of poor patient cooperation. At present, functional neuroimaging is used only in research settings.

American Psychiatric Association: Diagnostic and Statistical Manual of Mental Disorders, 5th Edition. Arlington, VA, American Psychiatric Association, 2013

Jacobson S, Jerrier H: EEG in delirium. Semin Clin Neuropsychiatry 5(2):86–92, 2000

Jacobson SA: Delirium in the elderly. Psychiatr Clin North Am 20(1):91–110, 1997

Diabetes mellitus	
Clinical diagnosis	Type 1 diabetes is an autoimmune disease usually diagnosed at or before adolescence. Although type 1 disease does involve insulin deficiency due to destruction of insulin-producing beta cells in the pancreas, the term "insulin-dependent" diabetes to describe this form is no longer in use, since type 2 diabetes can also develop into an insulin-dependent form. Symptoms of type 1 diabetes are like those of type 2 disease listed below, except that nausea, vomiting, and weight loss are also seen in type 1 disease.
	Type 2 diabetes is much more common than type 1 and has a high prevalence in the psychiatric population. Patients at risk of type 2 diabetes include those with hypertension, body mass index ≥25 or girth >88 cm (women) or 102 cm (men), hyperlipidemia (low high-density lipoprotein [HDL] or high triglycerides), vascular disease, family history in first-degree relative, high-risk ethnicity (e.g., African American, Latino), sedentary lifestyle, polycystic ovary syndrome, previous gestational diabetes, autoimmune disease (e.g., pernicious anemia, thyroid disease), or on diabeto-genic drugs (e.g., atypical antipsychotics, beta-blockers, or cortico-steroids).
	Symptoms of type 2 diabetes include polyuria, polydipsia, poly-phagia, fatigue, blurred vision, paresthesias, erectile dysfunction, and frequent or slow-healing infections.
Laboratory testing	Diabetes is diagnosed by the following laboratory findings: • Symptoms of diabetes plus random blood glucose ≥200 mg/dL (≥11.1 mmol/L) or • Fasting plasma glucose ≥126 mg/dL (≥7.0 mmol/L) or • Two-hour plasma glucose ≥200 mg/dL (≥11.1 mmol/L) during an oral glucose tolerance test. Test findings should be confirmed by repeat testing on a different day. Fasting plasma glucose is considered the best test for diag-nosing diabetes mellitus. Glucose tolerance testing is not recom-mended for routine care. Hemoglobin A_{1C} is not recommended to diagnose diabetes. In addition to testing patients who are symp-tomatic, active screening is recommended for patients over age 65 years, for those over 45 with one or more risk factors, and for those under 45 with two or more risk factors. For patients at risk, annual screening is recommended. For all patients over age 45, fasting glucose is recommended every 3 years.

American College of Endocrinology and American Diabetes Association Consensus statement on inpatient diabetes and glycemic control. Diabetes Care 29:1955–1962, 2006

Patel P, Macerollo A: Diabetes mellitus: diagnosis and screening. Am Fam Physician 81(7):863–870, 2010

Vijan S: Type 2 diabetes. Ann Intern Med 152:ITC31-15, quiz ITC316, 2010

Down syndrome (trisomy 21)

Clinical diagnosis	The risk of having a child with Down syndrome increases from 1 in 1,400 for women under age 25 to 1 in 100 for women age 40 years. Individuals with Down syndrome have characteristic physical features, including hypotonia, upwardly slanting palpebral fissures, midface depression, flat and wide nasal bridge, palmar simian crease, and short stature. Associated medical conditions include congenital heart disease, hearing problems, intestinal problems (e.g., small-bowel obstruction), celiac disease, eye problems (e.g., cataracts), thyroid abnormalities, skeletal problems, and very early onset Alzheimer's disease. Although most individuals with Down syndrome have IQs in the mildly to moderately low range, the symptoms can range from mild to severe. Language and motor development may be slow. In childhood, affected individuals are generally passive and affable, although they may be stubborn. Some individuals are hyperactive. Later in life, there is an increased risk of depression.
Laboratory testing	Four critical regions on chromosome 21 (DSCR1–4) have been described, and molecular markers for these regions and flanking regions enable the lab to identify cases of Down syndrome when more subtle abnormalities such as translocations are present or chromosomal abnormalities other than trisomy are involved. Genes outside the region on chromosome 21 (D21S55) may also contribute to the syndrome.
	Several tests are in common clinical use to determine the risk of Down syndrome in the developing fetus. In general, screening tests are low risk, but they are not definitive—they provide an estimate of the risk. Diagnostic tests introduce a risk of miscarriage, albeit small, but yield accurate information about whether the fetus has Down syndrome or other abnormalities.
	Screening tests include a blood test of *expanded alpha fetoprotein*, which is done between weeks 15 and 20 of pregnancy (ideally between weeks 16 and 18), and *nuchal translucency screening*, which is a high-resolution ultrasound of fetal neck tissue done between 11 and 14 weeks.
	Diagnostic tests include amniocentesis or chorionic villus sampling, both of which carry a risk of inducing abortion. *Amniocentesis* involves ultrasound-guided needle aspiration of amniotic fluid through the abdomen; it is usually performed between weeks 15 and 20 of pregnancy. *Chorionic villus sampling* involves ultrasound-guided biopsy of the placenta through the abdomen or cervix; it is usually performed between weeks 10 and 12. Results from the karyotype and other analyses from diagnostic tests are usually available after about 2 weeks. Diagnostic tests are usually reserved for pregnant women 35 years or older, for whom the risk of trisomy 21 in the fetus is higher. Fetal ultrasound can also be useful in the detection of birth defects in the fetus.

Eating disorders:
- **Anorexia nervosa**
- **Bulimia nervosa**

Clinical diagnosis	Anorexia nervosa
	• Restriction of energy intake relative to requirements, leading to a significantly low body weight
	• Intense fear of gaining weight or becoming fat, or persistent behavior that interferes with weight gain, even though at a significantly low weight
	• Disturbance in the way in which one's body weight or shape is experienced, undue influence of body weight or shape on self-evaluation, or persistent lack of recognition of the seriousness of the current low body weight
	• Restricting and binge-eating/purging types are specified
	Bulimia nervosa
	• Recurrent episodes of binge eating and recurrent inappropriate compensatory behaviors to prevent weight gain
	• Behaviors occurring at least once a week for 3 months
	• Self-evaluation unduly influenced by body shape and weight
Laboratory testing	For all patients with eating disorders:
	• Complete blood count with differential
	• Serum electrolytes
	• Blood urea nitrogen, creatinine
	• Liver function tests: aspartate transaminase, alanine transaminase, alkaline phosphatase
	• Thyroid-stimulating hormone (TSH); free T_4, T_3 if indicated
	• Erythrocyte sedimentation rate
	• Urinalysis
	Consider for malnourished and severely symptomatic patients:
	• Blood chemistries: calcium, magnesium, phosphorus
	• Complement component 3
	• Serum ferritin
	• Electrocardiogram
	• 24-hour urine for creatinine clearance

Eating disorders:
• **Anorexia nervosa**
• **Bulimia nervosa** *(continued)*

Laboratory testing *(continued)*	Osteopenia/osteoporosis screening:
	• Dual-energy X-ray absorptiometry (DEXA) scan for osteoporosis/osteopenia
	• Serum estradiol level in females
	• Serum testosterone level in males
	Consider for patients with persistent amenorrhea at normal weight:
	• Luteinizing hormone
	• Follicle-stimulating hormone
	• Beta-human chorionic gonadotropin
	• Prolactin
	For patients with suspected substance abuse:
	• Toxicology screen
	Consider for patients with cognitive deficits, neurological soft signs, unremitting course, or atypical features:
	• Brain magnetic resonance imaging or computed tomography
	For patients with suspected surreptitious vomiting:
	• Serum amylase (fractionated)
	For patients with suspected gastrointestinal bleeding:
	• Fecal occult blood testing
	For patients with suspected laxative abuse:
	• Stool or urine for bisacodyl, emodin, aloe-emodin, rhein

American Psychiatric Association: Diagnostic and Statistical Manual of Mental Disorders, 5th Edition. Arlington, VA, American Psychiatric Association, 2013

Rushing JM, Jones LE, Carney CP: Bulimia nervosa: a primary care review. Prim Care Companion J Clin Psychiatry 5(5):217–224, 2003

Treasure J, Claudino AM, Zucker N: Eating disorders. Lancet 375(9714):583–593, 2010

Yager J, Andersen AE: Clinical practice. Anorexia nervosa. N Engl J Med 353(14):1481–1488, 2005

Ethylene glycol poisoning	
Clinical diagnosis	Ethylene glycol is an odorless, sweet-tasting substance found in certain detergents, paints, de-icing products, brake fluid, and antifreeze. Ingestion of as little as 4 fluid ounces of ethylene glycol can kill an average-sized adult. Ethylene glycol can be accidentally ingested by children, intentionally taken in overdose, or abused as a substance in place of ethanol. With ingestion, the patient first appears intoxicated, with incoordination, nystagmus, slurred speech, and confusion. Nausea and vomiting can occur. Over time, metabolites of ethylene glycol accumulate, causing metabolic acidosis, tachycardia, hypertension, and hyperventilation. Hypocalcemia, QTc prolongation on electrocardiogram (ECG), congestive heart failure, and stupor progressing to coma may develop. The patient may die if untreated by this stage. If the patient survives, renal failure may occur, with acute tubular necrosis, hematuria, proteinuria, reduced urine output, and hyperkalemia. Renal failure can be reversed if supportive care is adequate; this may include months of hemodialysis.
Laboratory testing	The diagnosis can be made by the ethylene glycol level; toxicity is seen at levels >20 mg/dL. Some clinicians also check glycolic acid levels. Because the ethylene glycol assay is not available in all settings, the osmolal gap can be used in some cases as a proxy measure. A large osmolal gap supports the diagnosis in the patient with ingestion suspected on clinical grounds, but a normal gap does not exclude ingestion. In addition, other alcohols (e.g., methanol) or disorders such as lactic acidosis can also cause an increased gap. Other tests used in the diagnosis and management of ethylene glycol poisoning include the following: • Arterial blood gases • Comprehensive metabolic panel • Complete blood count • Blood ketones (to use in the assessment of osmolal gap) • Urine drug screen • Urinalysis (to look for calcium oxalate crystals) • Chest X ray • ECG • Head computed tomography (to detect cerebral edema)

Barceloux DG, Krenzelok EP, Olson K, et al: American Academy of Clinical Toxicology practice guidelines on the treatment of ethylene glycol poisoning. J Toxicol Clin Toxicol 37(5):537–560, 1999

Brent J: Current management of ethylene glycol poisoning. Drugs 61(7):979–988, 2001

Fatty liver disease (nonalcoholic)	
Clinical diagnosis	This is the most common cause of mildly increased liver function tests in the Western world, with a point prevalence of 23% among American adults. There is an increased risk of nonalcoholic fatty liver disease in patients with risk factors for the metabolic syndrome and insulin resistance, including obesity, diabetes, hyperlipidemia, and hypertension.
Laboratory testing	Laboratory abnormalities consistent with nonalcoholic fatty liver disease include the following: • Mild elevation in aspartate transaminase (AST) • Mild elevation in alanine transaminase (ALT) • Gamma-glutamyltransferase (GGT) up to three times the upper limit of normal in the absence of alcohol consumption

Ahmed MH: Biochemical markers: the road map for the diagnosis of nonalcoholic fatty liver disease. Am J Clin Pathol 127(1):20–22, 2007

Lidofsky SD: Nonalcoholic fatty liver disease: diagnosis and relation to metabolic syndrome and approach to treatment. Curr Diab Rep 8(1):25–30, 2008

Myers RP: Noninvasive diagnosis of nonalcoholic fatty liver disease. Ann Hepatol 8 (Suppl 1):S25–S33, 2009

Folate deficiency	
Clinical diagnosis	Folate deficiency occurs in the clinical setting of malnutrition, alcoholism, or malabsorption, or with the use of anticonvulsant drugs, in pregnancy, with reticulocytosis after vitamin B_{12} replacement, or with hemodialysis. Symptoms resemble those of vitamin B_{12} deficiency, and include the following: • Dementia • Peripheral neuropathy (decreased vibration sense in lower extremities) • Ataxia • Positive Romberg test • Paraplegia with extensor plantar responses and deep tendon reflex abnormalities (hyporeflexia or hyperreflexia)
Laboratory testing	• A macrocytic anemia is seen, with hypersegmented neutrophils and macro-ovalocytes. • Red blood cell folate is superior to serum folate because it is a better reflection of tissue levels. Plasma homocysteine, which is even more sensitive, is increased in folate deficiency but is nonspecific. • Before folate therapy is initiated, B_{12} deficiency should be excluded with a normal B_{12} level and a normal methylmalonic acid level. These deficiencies may occur in tandem, and replacement of folate alone may result in clinical worsening. • To monitor the effectiveness of folate replacement, a complete blood count (CBC) should be performed after 2 weeks to document increase in hemoglobin and decrease in mean corpuscular volume; another CBC should be performed after 8 weeks to document resolution of anemia. • Long-term folate replacement is not necessary unless the cause persists (e.g., malnutrition); long-term monitoring is usually not needed.

Lerner V, Kanevsky M, Dwolatzky T, et al: Vitamin B_{12} and folate serum levels in newly admitted psychiatric patients. Clin Nutr 25(1):60–67, 2006

Tolmunen T, Voutilainen S, Hintikka J, et al: Dietary folate and depressive symptoms are associated in middle-aged Finnish men. J Nutr 133(10):3233–3236, 2003

Triantafyllou NI, Nikolaou C, Boufidou F, et al: Folate and vitamin B_{12} levels in levodopa-treated Parkinson's disease patients: their relationship to clinical manifestations, mood and cognition. Parkinsonism Relat Disord 14(4):321–325, 2008

Generalized anxiety disorder (GAD)	
Clinical diagnosis	GAD is characterized by excessive anxiety and worry about a number of events or activities, occurring more days than not for at least 6 months. The individual has difficulty controlling the worry. The anxiety and worry are associated with three or more of the following symptoms (only one symptom in children): restlessness (feeling "keyed up" or "on edge"), being easily fatigued, difficulty concentrating, irritability, muscle tension, and/or sleep disturbance. The signs and symptoms cause significant distress or impairment in function. The disturbance is not attributable to the physiological effects of a substance or another medical condition, and is not better explained by another mental disorder.
Laboratory testing	The basic laboratory workup for GAD includes only a metabolic panel (basic or comprehensive) to check calcium and glucose levels, and thyroid-stimulating hormone. Further testing may be indicated to exclude medical conditions causing or contributing to anxiety. Depending on patient characteristics and history, further evaluation might include one or more of the following: • Electrocardiogram, Holter monitoring, cardiac stress testing, and/or echocardiogram • Chest X ray, pulmonary function tests, and/or arterial blood gases • Gamma-glutamyltransferase (GGT) with or without carbohydrate-deficient transferrin (%CDT) for suspicion of covert drinking • Plasma free metanephrines • Urine porphyrin precursors • Pulmonary computed tomography scan • Electroencephalogram

American Psychiatric Association: Diagnostic and Statistical Manual of Mental Disorders, 5th Edition. Arlington, VA, American Psychiatric Association, 2013

Hepatic encephalopathy (HE)

Clinical diagnosis	HE is a cognitive disorder that can occur in a patient with liver failure. Onset may be acute or subacute, or the condition may be present chronically (e.g., in cirrhosis). With acute onset, the presentation is one of delirium, with disturbance in consciousness, day/night reversal, and cognitive impairment that includes inattention, disorientation, executive dysfunction, visuospatial impairment, and acalculia, among other impairments. Asterixis is often seen, and seizures may occur. In severe cases, cerebral edema and brain herniation may ensue. Chronic hyperammonemia has less florid effects because of compensatory effects in ammonia metabolism and dampening of excitatory effects on the brain. The patient appears slow and lethargic, with a variable degree of dementia with subcortical features. Mostly for purposes of transplant care, HE is graded and typed as follows: • Grade 1 (minimal HE)—trivial lack of awareness, euphoria or anxiety, reduced attention span, impaired performance on an addition task • Grade 2—lethargy, apathy, minimal disorientation to time or place, subtle personality change, inappropriate behavior, impaired performance on a subtraction task • Grade 3—somnolence to semistupor, responsive to verbal stimuli, confusion, gross disorientation • Grade 4—coma (unresponsive to verbal or noxious stimuli) • Type A—acute HE with liver failure • Type B—bypass (portosystemic shunting without liver disease) • Type C—cirrhosis
Laboratory testing	The ammonia level is elevated, but the degree of elevation does not correlate with the severity of encephalopathy except in acute HE. (See the Ammonia [NH_3] entry in Chapter 1, "Laboratory Tests.") The electroencephalogram shows generalized slowing, slowing of the posterior dominant frequency, triphasic waves, and in some cases, epileptiform activity. Even in patients with known underlying liver disease, the following possible precipitants should be investigated: • Hyponatremia • Hypokalemia • Alkalosis • Dehydration

Hepatic encephalopathy (HE) *(continued)*	
Laboratory testing *(continued)*	• Hypoglycemia • Renal insufficiency • Infection (e.g., spontaneous bacterial peritonitis) • Blood in the gastrointestinal tract • Use of alcohol or certain drugs, such as benzodiazepines or opioids

Cohn RM, Roth KS: Hyperammonemia, bane of the brain. Clin Pediatr (Phila) 43(8):683–689, 2004

Kundra A, Jain A, Banga A, et al: Evaluation of plasma ammonia levels in patients with acute liver failure and chronic liver disease and its correlation with the severity of hepatic encephalopathy and clinical features of raised intracranial tension. Clin Biochem 38(8):696–699, 2005

Record CO: Neurochemistry of hepatic encephalopathy. Gut 32(11):1261–1263, 1991

Hepatitis (viral)	
Clinical diagnosis	Hepatitis A, B, C, D, and E are caused by viruses that lead to hepatocellular disease, with liver injury, inflammation, and necrosis. In the United States, 95% of cases are accounted for by hepatitis A, B, and C viruses. Hepatitis A and E are transmitted through the fecal-oral route, whereas hepatitis B, C, and D are transmitted through body fluids. Sexual exposure is a common mode of transmission for hepatitis B but is rare for hepatitis C. Needle sharing is the most common mode of transmission for hepatitis C, but it also can transmit hepatitis B. Hepatitis B has high seroprevalence among methadone clinic patients. Blood transfusion received before 1992 was a risk factor for hepatitis C. Vertical transmission from mother to infant occurs with hepatitis B and C. Hepatitis A, which can be contracted from contaminated food, is generally a mild, self-limited disease. Hepatitis B, C, and D may become chronic._x000D_ Hepatitis can be asymptomatic, manifested only by a slight rise in aspartate transaminase (AST) and alanine transaminase (ALT) levels. When symptoms are present, the most common one is fatigue, which is worse later in the day after activity, but which may be intermittent and of varying severity. Other symptoms include nausea, right upper quadrant pain, anorexia, pruritis, and jaundice. In many patients, the physical exam is normal, unless the disease is acute or fairly advanced.

Laboratory testing	General evaluation of liver disease: AST, ALT, alkaline phosphatase (ALP), bilirubin (total and direct), albumin, and prothrombin time. On the basis of these tests, hepatocellular versus cholestatic disease can be diagnosed, and it can be determined whether the process is acute or chronic and whether cirrhosis or hepatic failure is present.
	
	Type of viral hepatitis can be determined by serology:
	
	• Hepatitis A: anti-HAV immunoglobulin M (IgM)
	
	• Hepatitis B:
	  • Acute—HbsAg and anti-HBc IgM
	  • Chronic—HbsAg and HbeAg and/or HBV DNA
	
	• Hepatitis C: anti-HCV and HCV RNA
	
	• Hepatitis D (delta): HbsAg and anti-HDV
	
	• Hepatitis E: anti-HEV
	
	Diagnostic imaging (ultrasonography, computed tomography, and/or magnetic resonance imaging) may be needed, although none of these methods can accurately detect cirrhosis.

Bart G, Piccolo P, Zhang L, et al: Markers for hepatitis A, B and C in methadone maintained patients: an unexpectedly high co-infection with silent hepatitis B. Addiction 103(4):681–686, 2008

Lin YH, Wang Y, Loua A, et al: Evaluation of a new hepatitis B virus surface antigen rapid test with improved sensitivity. J Clin Microbiol 46(10):3319–3324, 2008

National Institutes of Health Consensus Statement on Management of Hepatitis C: 2002. NIH Consens State Sci Statements, 19:1–46, 2002

HIV/AIDS	
Clinical diagnosis	Most HIV infections in the United States are HIV-1; HIV-2 is endemic to West Africa. With infection, the virus localizes to lymphoid tissues, infecting CD4+ helper cells and T-cell lymphocytes. A viremia occurs, which can be intense and rapid. Signs and symptoms of this acute retroviral syndrome typically include the following: • Fever • Fatigue • Rash • Headache • Lymphadenopathy • Pharyngitis • Myalgias • Nausea, vomiting, and/or diarrhea • Night sweats Cranial nerve palsies may also be seen with seroconversion, as signs of aseptic meningitis. In rare cases, encephalitis can occur. Transverse myelitis and peripheral polyneuropathy can also be seen. The symptoms of the acute syndrome resolve within days to weeks. When viremia clears, the patient enters a latent stage without clinical symptoms. The following are seen with progression to AIDS in treated or untreated patients: • CD4+<2,000 cells/µL • Opportunistic infections • Malignancies (Kaposi sarcoma, non-Hodgkin lymphoma, invasive cervical cancer, primary brain non-Hodgkin lymphoma) • Chronic metabolic derangements (impaired glucose tolerance, dyslipidemia, lipodystrophy)
Laboratory testing	The U.S. Preventive Services Task Force recommends screening for HIV infection in adolescents and adults ages 15–65 years. Younger adolescents and older adults who are at increased risk also should be screened. One-time screening of adolescent and adult patients is recommended to identify those already HIV-positive, with repeated screening of those known to be at risk for HIV infection, those actively engaged in risky behaviors, and those who live or receive medical care in a high-prevalence setting.

HIV/AIDS *(continued)*	
Laboratory testing *(continued)*	It may be reasonable to rescreen groups at very high risk for new HIV infection at least annually and individuals at increased risk at somewhat longer intervals (e.g., 3–5 years). Routine rescreening may not be necessary for individuals who have not been at increased risk since they were found to be HIV-negative. Women screened during a previous pregnancy should be rescreened in subsequent pregnancies.
	Screening tests become positive 3–5 weeks after infection.
	The conventional serum test for diagnosing HIV infection is the repeatedly reactive immunoassay followed by confirmatory Western blot or immunofluorescent assay. The test is highly accurate (sensitivity and specificity, >99.5%), and results are available within 1–2 days from most commercial laboratories.
	Rapid HIV testing may use either blood or oral fluid specimens and can provide results in 5–40 minutes. The sensitivity and specificity of the rapid test also are both >99.5%; however, initial positive results require confirmation with conventional methods.
	Other U.S. Food and Drug Administration–approved tests for detection and confirmation of HIV infection include combination tests (for p24 antigen and HIV antibodies) and qualitative HIV-1 RNA.
	Treatment is monitored using quantitative viral load, CD4$^+$ count, and drug resistance testing (genotyping).

Price RW, Epstein LG, Becker JT, et al: Biomarkers of HIV-1 CNS infection and injury. Neurology 69:1781–1788, 2007

Syed Iqbal H, Balakrishnan P, Murugavel KG, et al: Performance characteristics of a new rapid immunochromatographic test for the detection of antibodies to human immunodeficiency virus (HIV) types 1 and 2. J Clin Lab Anal 22(3):178–185, 2008

U.S. Preventive Services Task Force: Screening for HIV: recommendation statement. Ann Intern Med 143(1):32–37, 2005

Hydrocephalus	
Clinical diagnosis	When the path of cerebrospinal fluid (CSF) circulation is blocked such that absorption is impaired, ventricular pressure builds up proximal to the block and the ventricles become dilated, a condition known as hydrocephalus. When the block is inside the ventricular system, noncommunicating hydrocephalus results, meaning that the CSF does not continue to flow or "communicate" with the rest of the subarachnoid space, such as that surrounding the spinal cord. When the block is outside the ventricular system, such as over the cerebral convexities in the arachnoid villi, communicating hydrocephalus results.
	Normal-pressure hydrocephalus (NPH) is a chronic form of communicating hydrocephalus. Patients with chronic, slowly developing hydrocephalus may show the classic NPH triad of dementia, ataxia, and urinary incontinence. The dementia is characterized by memory impairment, motor and cognitive slowing, and apathy or indifference. Rarely, delusional thinking is prominent. The ataxia is actually a gait apraxia in which movement is stiff and hesitant and feet appear to be stuck to the floor ("magnetic" gait). Urinary urgency may be reported rather than frank incontinence. Hyperreflexia and extensor plantar responses may be seen. Primitive reflexes (grasp and snout) may be present.
	Patients with acute hydrocephalus present *in extremis*, with headache, vomiting, and stupor. Papilledema may be noted. These patients are at risk of rapid progression to coma and death. This form of hydrocephalus is usually a noncommunicating form, with complete or nearly complete obstruction of flow.
	Hydrocephalus *ex vacuo* occurs when ventricles expand with atrophy of brain tissue, such as with Alzheimer's disease. In this case, intracranial pressure is not increased.
Laboratory testing	• Both computed tomography (CT) and magnetic resonance imaging (MRI) will demonstrate the ventricular enlargement, but MRI is superior to CT in identifying the site of obstruction.
	• Transependymal fluid shift is seen as hypodense areas on CT and hyperintense areas on MRI surrounding the ventricles.
	• In distinguishing true hydrocephalus from hydrocephalus *ex vacuo*, which can occur in patients with dementia of other etiologies, the following findings are considered:
	• Ventricular enlargement greater than sulcal enlargement (seen with cortical atrophy) supports true hydrocephalus with increased pressure.
	• T2 hyperintensities surrounding the lateral ventricles consistent with transependymal extravasation of CSF support true hydrocephalus.

Factora R, Luciano M: When to consider normal pressure hydrocephalus in the patient with gait disturbance. Geriatrics 63(2):32–37, 2008
Garton HJ, Piatt JH Jr: Hydrocephalus. Pediatr Clin North Am 51(2):305–325, 2004

Hyperthyroidism	
Clinical diagnosis	Hyperthyroidism occurs in women more frequently than in men. It can occur in the context of Graves disease (onset in third or fourth decade; most common cause of hyperthyroidism), Hashimoto thyroiditis (onset in middle age), multinodular goiter (onset in older age), or pregnancy.

Physical signs and symptoms include the following:

- Tachycardia
- Weight loss despite increased appetite and eating
- Widened palpebral fissures ("bug eyes")
- Eye irritation
- Heat intolerance, sweating
- Tremors (fine distal hand)
- Chorea
- Hyperactive deep tendon reflexes
- Diarrhea or increased frequency of bowel movements
- Alopecia
- Menstrual irregularities in women
- Erectile dysfunction in men

Psychiatric signs and symptoms include the following:

- Depression (more common than anxiety)
- Anxiety
- Mania or hypomania
- Psychosis
- Delirium
- Restlessness, agitation
- Insomnia
- Fatigue

The syndrome of apathetic hyperthyroidism affects primarily geriatric patients and includes symptoms of lethargy, tachycardia, atrial fibrillation, heart failure, and cognitive impairment severe enough to warrant a diagnosis of dementia.

Thyroid storm involves the hyperacute development of symptoms in a patient with untreated hyperthyroidism who becomes medically ill or undergoes surgery. Severe symptoms are seen, along with fever and delirium.

Hyperthyroidism *(continued)*

Laboratory testing	• First check thyroid-stimulating hormone (TSH); many clinicians will also check free thyroxine (T_4) at this time. • If TSH is low (or if clinical suspicion is high), check free T_4. • If free T_4 is high, the patient has hyperthyroidism. • Further evaluation may involve checking the thyroid antibodies TPO, TRAb, and TSI (thyroid peroxidase, TSH receptor antibody, and thyroid-stimulating immunoglobulin) or radioiodine uptake of the thyroid.

Iglesias P, Dévora O, García J, et al: Severe hyperthyroidism: aetiology, clinical features and treatment outcome. Clin Endocrinol (Oxf) 72(4):551–557, 2010

Shulman DI, Muhar I, Jorgensen EV, et al: Autoimmune hyperthyroidism in prepubertal children and adolescents: comparison of clinical and biochemical features at diagnosis and responses to medical therapy. Thyroid 7(5):755–760, 1997

Spaulding SW, Lippes H: Hyperthyroidism. Causes, clinical features, and diagnosis. Med Clin North Am 69(5):937–951, 1985

Hypothyroidism	
Clinical diagnosis	Risk of hypothyroidism is greater for females and increases with age. Risk is also associated with the following drugs: amiodarone, gonadal steroid hormones, glucocorticoids, furosemide, lithium, levodopa, neuroleptics, phenytoin, and propranolol, among others. Onset of hypothyroidism is usually insidious. Signs and symptoms include the following: • Fatigue • Depression • Psychosis ("myxedema madness") in about 10% • Memory impairment • Cold intolerance • Weight gain • Alopecia • Bradycardia • Dry skin • Skin thickening (myxedema), often most apparent on face, legs, and dorsum of hands and feet • Carpal tunnel syndrome • Coma In pregnancy, hypothyroidism is associated with symptoms of bradycardia, low energy, inappropriate weight gain, constipation, goiter, and cold intolerance. The fetus may be adversely affected.
Laboratory testing	• First check thyroid-stimulating hormone (TSH); many clinicians will also check free thyroxine (T_4) at this time. • If TSH is high (or if clinical suspicion is high), check free thyroxine (T_4). • If free T_4 is low, the patient is hypothyroid. Differential diagnosis includes primary hypothyroidism, euthyroid sick syndrome, transient thyroiditis, and iatrogenic cause (e.g., thyroid ablation). • If free T_4 is normal, further workup might include thyroid antibodies to diagnose possible autoimmune thyroid disease.

Baskin HJ, Cobin RH, Duick DS, et al; American Association of Clinical Endocrinologists: American Association of Clinical Endocrinologists medical guidelines for clinical practice for the evaluation and treatment of hyperthyroidism and hypothyroidism. Endocr Pract 8(6):457–469, 2002
Roberts CG, Ladenson PW: Hypothyroidism. Lancet 363(9411):793–803, 2004
Surks MI, Ortiz E, Daniels GH, et al: Subclinical thyroid disease: scientific review and guidelines for diagnosis and management. JAMA 291(2):228–238, 2004

Intellectual disability	
Clinical diagnosis	Intellectual disability is identified by the presence of deficits in intellectual functions and adaptive functioning with onset during the developmental period. Intellectual functions include reasoning, problem solving, planning, abstract thinking, judgment, academic learning, and learning from experience. Deficits in these functions are confirmed by clinical assessment and standardized intelligence testing. Deficits in adaptive functioning result in failure to meet developmental and sociocultural standards for personal independence and social responsibility. Without ongoing support, the adaptive deficits limit functioning in one or more activities of daily living. Severity (mild, moderate, severe, profound) is determined by comparison to conceptual, social, and practical domain benchmarks described in DSM-5 rather than IQ cutoff scores.
Laboratory testing	The laboratory evaluation may involve testing for conditions such as the following: • Inborn errors of metabolism with autosomal recessive inheritance (e.g., Tay-Sachs disease) • Single-gene abnormalities with Mendelian inheritance and variable expression (e.g., tuberous sclerosis) • Chromosomal aberrations (fragile X syndrome) • Down syndrome due to trisomy 21 • Lead poisoning • Early traumatic brain injury Testing is more likely to reveal an etiology when mental retardation is severe or profound.

American Psychiatric Association: Diagnostic and Statistical Manual of Mental Disorders, 5th Edition. Arlington, VA, American Psychiatric Association, 2013

Lead poisoning

Clinical diagnosis	Acute ingestion of a large amount of lead (e.g., a patient with pica eating lead chips) is associated with colicky abdominal pain, a metallic taste, and then a florid delirium termed *lead encephalopathy*. Acute lead poisoning can be fatal. Those who survive acute poisoning are usually left with cognitive and motor deficits. In adults, chronic low-level lead exposure typically results in mild cognitive impairment and a peripheral motor neuropathy with wrist and foot drop. These patients may or may not report abdominal pain or metallic taste. Chronic low-level exposure has cumulative effects and may go unnoticed until the patient presents with dementia, clear motor deficits, or kidney failure. Other signs and symptoms of lead poisoning in adults include the following: • Fatigue • Weakness • Mood changes (depression, irritability) • Personality changes (apathy) • Memory problems • Headaches • Tremors • Seizures • Coma • Nausea, vomiting, and/or diarrhea • Loss of appetite and weight loss • Anemia • Reproductive failure Signs and symptoms that may occur in infants and children include the following: • Behavioral problems • Developmental delays • Growth failure • Cognitive impairment and academic problems • Hearing loss • Sleep problems In some cases, infants and children are asymptomatic during the time of exposure but still suffer permanent brain damage.

Lead poisoning *(continued)*	
Laboratory testing	Lead level can be measured in blood or 24-hour urine, but blood is the specimen of choice. See lab report for reference range.

Critical values of lead in blood:

- Pregnant women: ≥10 µg/dL
- Children: >20 µg/dL
- Adults: >45 µg/dL
- Medical emergency (any age): >70 µg/dL

Reference interval for 24-hour urine lead: 0–31 µg/dL

Zinc protoporphyrin concentration was once used to screen for lead exposure in children, but it has been found to be unreliable at lead concentrations <250 µg/L (0.40 µmol/L) and is no longer recommended for this application.

Patients with elevated lead levels should be tested for anemia and iron deficiency, because lead interferes with iron absorption. |

Brewster UC, Perazella MA: A review of chronic lead intoxication: an unrecognized cause of chronic kidney disease. Am J Med Sci 327(6):341–347, 2004

Brown JS: Environmental and Chemical Toxins and Psychiatric Illness. Washington, DC, American Psychiatric Publishing, 2002

Wu AHB: Tietz Clinical Guide to Laboratory Tests, 4th Edition. St. Louis, MO, WB Saunders, 2006

Major depressive episode	
Clinical diagnosis	This condition is characterized by five or more of the following symptoms* present nearly every day during the same 2-week period and representing a change from previous function: • Depressed mood (can be irritable mood in children and adolescents) • Marked loss of interest or pleasure in activities • Change in appetite or weight (can be failure to make expected weight gains in children) • Insomnia or hypersomnia • Psychomotor agitation or retardation • Fatigue or loss of energy • Feelings of worthlessness or excessive guilt • Reduced ability to think, concentrate, or make decisions • Recurrent thoughts of death, recurrent suicidal ideation, or suicide attempt or specific plan for suicide *At least one of the symptoms must be either depressed mood or loss of interest or pleasure. The symptoms cause significant distress or impairment of function, and are not attributable to the effects of a substance or to another medical condition.
Laboratory testing	The following laboratory tests should be considered to exclude secondary depression, precipitants or contributors to idiopathic depression, and comorbid conditions and/or to help guide treatment: • Comprehensive metabolic panel • Complete blood count with differential and platelets • Folate level • Urinalysis • Urine toxic screen • Thyroid-stimulating hormone (TSH) • Rapid plasma reagin (RPR) • HIV testing in selected cases • Blood alcohol level in selected cases • Medication levels (for tricyclics or mood stabilizers) • Urine pregnancy testing, if indicated • Magnetic resonance imaging or electroencephalogram if there is suspicion of a structural abnormality or seizures

American Psychiatric Association: Diagnostic and Statistical Manual of Mental Disorders, 5th Edition. Arlington, VA, American Psychiatric Association, 2013

Manic episode	
Clinical diagnosis	Manic episode is characterized by a distinct period of abnormally and persistently elevated, expansive, or irritable mood and abnormally and persistently increased activity or energy, lasting at least 1 week and present most of the day, nearly every day (or any duration if hospitalization is necessary). During this period, three or more of the following symptoms are present (four or more symptoms if the mood is only irritable): • Grandiosity • Decreased need for sleep • Pressured speech or talkativeness • Flight of ideas or racing thoughts • Distractibility • Increase in goal-directed activity or psychomotor agitation • Excessive involvement in activities that have a high potential for painful consequences The symptoms cause significant impairment of function or necessitate hospitalization, or include psychotic features. The symptoms are not attributable to the physiological effects of a substance or to another medical condition. A full manic episode that emerges during antidepressant treatment and persists at a fully syndromal level beyond the physiological effects of that treatment is sufficient evidence for a manic episode.
Laboratory testing	The following laboratory tests should be considered to exclude secondary mania, precipitants or contributors to idiopathic mania, and comorbid conditions and/or to help guide treatment: • Comprehensive metabolic panel • Complete blood count with differential and platelets • Urinalysis • Thyroid-stimulating hormone (TSH) • Rapid plasma reagin (RPR)

Manic episode *(continued)*	
Laboratory testing *(continued)*	In the presence of risk factors or suggestive history, the following tests also should be considered: • Urine toxicology • HIV testing • Blood alcohol level • Urine pregnancy testing • Electroencephalogram (to exclude epileptiform activity) • Brain magnetic resonance imaging or head computed tomography

American Psychiatric Association: Practice Guidelines for the Treatment of Psychiatric Disorders. Washington, DC, American Psychiatric Association, 2000

American Psychiatric Association: Diagnostic and Statistical Manual of Mental Disorders, 5th Edition. Arlington, VA, American Psychiatric Association, 2013

Metabolic syndrome	
Clinical diagnosis	Patients at risk of the metabolic syndrome include those treated with the psychotropic medications associated with weight gain, including the atypical antipsychotics (especially clozapine and olanzapine), all antidepressants except possibly bupropion, and mood stabilizers. The syndrome is defined by specific physical and laboratory abnormalities, as noted below.
Laboratory testing	Metabolic syndrome is defined by three or more of the following: • Waist circumference in males >40 inches (>102 cm); in females >35 inches (>88 cm) • Fasting glucose ≥100 mg/dL • Blood pressure ≥130/85 • Triglycerides ≥150 mg/dL • High-density lipoprotein (HDL) cholesterol in males <40 mg/dL; in females <50 mg/dL

Olufadi R, Byrne CD: Clinical and laboratory diagnosis of the metabolic syndrome. J Clin Pathol 61(6):697–706, 2008

Methanol poisoning

Clinical diagnosis	Methanol is an extremely toxic substance found in antifreeze, shellac, varnish, paint thinner, fuel additives, de-icing fluids, and copy machine fluids. It may be ingested accidentally, taken in overdose intentionally, or abused by alcoholics without access to ethanol. As little as 2 tablespoons can be lethal for a child, and 2 fluid ounces for an adult. The prognosis with poisoning depends on the amount ingested and how soon treatment is administered.
	The most common presenting symptoms are visual disturbances (photophobia, blurring, decreased acuity) and abdominal pain (with or without pancreatitis). Cognitive changes are present within the first 24 hours and may be the only abnormalities for several days if the patient has also ingested ethanol. Symptoms worsen as formic acid is generated from methanol. Seizures can occur. Confusion, stupor, and coma often develop. Permanent visual impairment is seen in up to 18% of affected patients. A rare sequel is putaminal necrosis, with parkinsonian symptoms (rigidity, tremor, masked facies, and monotonous speech). Respiratory failure and/or cardiac arrest may occur. Survivors may be blind or neurologically impaired.
Laboratory testing	A serum methanol level >20 mg/dL soon after ingestion is an indication for treatment with an antidote such as ethanol or fomepizole. However, blood methanol is measured by gas chromatography in specialty labs, so this test is not universally available, and it may take days for results to return. In the absence of blood methanol measurements, the serum osmolal gap can be used to confirm the clinical diagnosis and to guide management.
	Other laboratory abnormalities include blood gases and chemistries indicating metabolic acidosis, abnormal liver function test results, and elevated lipase indicating pancreatitis.

Kraut JA, Kurtz I: Toxic alcohol ingestions: clinical features, diagnosis, and management. Clin J Am Soc Nephrol 3(1):208–225, 2008

Neuroleptic malignant syndrome (NMS)

Clinical diagnosis	Patients at risk of NMS include those with dehydration or infection, those with neurological diseases such as Parkinson's disease, and those treated with neuroleptic medications or rapidly withdrawn from dopamine agonists (e.g., levodopa or ropinirole). Genetic factors may have a role.
	Symptoms come on acutely and are fully developed within 24–48 hours. Signs and symptoms include the following:
	• Fever
	• Muscle rigidity (lead pipe or cogwheel)
	• Fluctuating consciousness, delirium, catatonia
	• Autonomic instability: diaphoresis, pallor or flushing, tachycardia, hypertension, hypotension, cardiac dysrhythmia, tachypnea, dyspnea, and urinary incontinence
	• Movement abnormalities: coarse tremor, bradykinesia, dystonia (opisthotonos, blepharospasm, oculogyric crisis, or trismus), chorea, and oral-buccal dyskinesias resembling tardive dyskinesia
	Complications include pneumonia, pulmonary embolism, cardiac arrest or dysrhythmia, disseminated intravascular coagulation, rhabdomyolysis, and renal failure. The syndrome can be fatal.
Laboratory testing	• Elevated creatine kinase (of 200 U/L to >100,000 U/L)
	• Leukocytosis, often with left shift
	• Liver function test abnormalities (aspartate transaminase [AST] and alanine transaminase [ALT] elevation)
	• Myoglobinuria

Rosebush PI, Anglin RE, Richards C, et al: Neuroleptic malignant syndrome and the acute phase response. J Clin Psychopharmacol 28(4):459–461, 2008

Strawn JR, Keck PE Jr, Caroff SN: Neuroleptic malignant syndrome. Am J Psychiatry 164(6):870–876, 2007

Obsessive-compulsive disorder (OCD)	
Clinical diagnosis	OCD is characterized by the presence of obsessions, compulsions, or both. Obsessions are recurrent and persistent thoughts, urges, or images that are experienced, at some time during the disturbance, as intrusive and unwanted and that in most individuals cause marked anxiety or distress. The individual attempts to ignore or suppress such thoughts, urges, or images or to neutralize them with some other thought or action (i.e., by performing a compulsion). Compulsions are repetitive behaviors (e.g., hand washing, ordering, checking) or mental acts (e.g., praying, counting, repeating words silently) that the individual feels driven to perform in response to an obsession, or according to rules that must be applied rigidly. The behaviors or mental acts are aimed at preventing or reducing anxiety or distress or preventing some dreaded event or situation; however, these behaviors or mental acts are not connected in a realistic way with what they are designed to neutralize or prevent or are clearly excessive. The obsessions or compulsions are time-consuming (e.g., take more than 1 hour per day) or cause clinically significant distress or impairment in functioning. The content of the obsessions or compulsions is not restricted to the symptoms of another mental disorder. Insight is variable. The affected patient may have a current or past history of a tic disorder.
Laboratory testing	The basic laboratory workup for anxiety includes only a metabolic panel (basic metabolic panel or comprehensive metabolic panel) to check calcium and glucose levels, and thyroid-stimulating hormone. Depending on patient characteristics and history, other elements of the evaluation might include one or more of the following: • Electrocardiogram, Holter monitoring, cardiac stress testing, and/or echocardiogram • Chest X ray, pulmonary function tests, and/or arterial blood gases • Gamma-glutamyltransferase (GGT) with or without carbohydrate-deficient transferrin (%CDT) for suspicion of covert drinking • Plasma free metanephrines • Urine porphyrin precursors • Pulmonary computed tomography scan • Electroencephalogram Patients who are to be started on certain psychotropic medications to treat OCD will require screening and monitoring lab tests as outlined in Chapter 3, "Psychotropic Medications."

American Psychiatric Association: Diagnostic and Statistical Manual of Mental Disorders, 5th Edition. Arlington, VA, American Psychiatric Association, 2013

Panic attack; panic disorder

Clinical diagnosis	A *panic attack* is characterized by an abrupt surge of intense fear or intense discomfort that reaches a peak within minutes, and during which time four or more of the following symptoms occur: • Palpitations, pounding heart, or accelerated heart rate • Sweating • Trembling or shaking • Sensations of shortness of breath or smothering • Feelings of choking • Chest pain or discomfort • Nausea or abdominal distress • Feeling dizzy, unsteady, lightheaded, or faint • Chills or heat sensations • Paresthesias (numbness or tingling sensations) • Derealization (feelings of unreality) or depersonalization (being detached from oneself) • Fear of losing control or "going crazy" • Fear of dying *Panic disorder* is defined by recurrent, unexpected panic attacks accompanied by persistent concern or worry about additional panic attacks or their consequences and/or significant maladaptive change in behavior such as avoidance. Panic disorder is a primary condition (i.e., the panic attacks are not attributable to the physiological effects of a substance or another medical condition, and are not restricted to the symptoms of another mental disorder).
Laboratory testing	Isolated panic attacks may not require laboratory workup. For recurrent panic attacks, a metabolic panel (basic or comprehensive) to check calcium and glucose levels, and thyroid function testing to check thyroid-stimulating hormone are recommended. Depending on patient characteristics and history, other elements of the evaluation might include one or more of the following: • Electrocardiogram, Holter monitoring, cardiac stress testing, and/or echocardiogram • Chest X ray, pulmonary function tests, and/or arterial blood gases • Urine drug screening (especially for cannabis and hallucinogens)

Panic attack; panic disorder *(continued)*	
Laboratory testing *(continued)*	• Gamma-glutamyltransferase (GGT) with or without carbohydrate-deficient transferrin (%CDT) for suspicion of covert drinking
	• Plasma free metanephrines to exclude pheochromocytoma
	• Urine porphyrin precursors
	• Pulmonary computed tomography scan
	• Electroencephalogram to exclude seizures

American Psychiatric Association: Diagnostic and Statistical Manual of Mental Disorders, 5th Edition. Arlington, VA, American Psychiatric Association, 2013

Pica	
Clinical diagnosis	Pica is characterized by persistent eating of nonnutritive, nonfood substances over a period of at least 1 month, where the eating of these substances is inappropriate to the developmental level of the individual and is not part of a culturally supported or socially normative practice. If the behavior occurs in the context of another mental disorder (e.g., intellectual disability, autism spectrum disorder, schizophrenia), it must be sufficiently severe to warrant additional clinical attention.
Laboratory testing	• Complete blood count to diagnose anemia • Serum iron level (often low) • Serum zinc level (often low) • Lead level in cases where ingested material includes paint or other lead-containing substances • Barium X ray or endoscopy to identify swallowed objects or gastric bezoar

American Psychiatric Association: Diagnostic and Statistical Manual of Mental Disorders, 5th Edition. Arlington, VA, American Psychiatric Association, 2013

Polydipsia (psychogenic)	
Clinical diagnosis	Patients at risk of psychogenic polydipsia include those with schizophrenia or developmental disabilities. Signs and symptoms include the following: • Excessive water intake • Polyuria • Seizures (severe cases) • Cardiac arrest (severe cases) Cerebral edema with herniation has been reported. The syndrome can be fatal. A milder form of overdrinking—"habit polydipsia"—may be seen in other psychiatric populations and results in less severe symptoms.
Laboratory testing	The following laboratory abnormalities are seen in polydipsia: • Hyponatremia • Low serum and urine osmolality • Low serum vasopressin Nonsuppression on the dexamethasone suppression test has been described, but this test is not routinely used to diagnose polydipsia.

Dundas B, Harris M, Narasimhan M: Psychogenic polydipsia review: etiology, differential, and treatment. Curr Psychiatry Rep 9(3):236–241, 2007

Leiken SJ, Caplan H: Psychogenic polydipsia. Am J Psychiatry 123(12):1573–1576, 1967

Psychotic disorder due to another medical condition	
Clinical diagnosis	This syndrome is one of prominent hallucinations or delusions occurring in a patient with a clear sensorium (not delirious). The symptoms are not psychologically mediated, but instead are the direct effects of a substance or medical condition. Modality of hallucinations may suggest the area of the brain affected (e.g., olfactory with complex partial seizures arising from temporal lobes or visual with occipital lobe tumors), but this is less true for delusions.
	Patients at risk include those with substance abuse; those taking certain medications (levodopa or other Parkinson's disease drugs, sympathomimetics); those with known epilepsy, traumatic brain injury, stroke, or degenerative brain disease; and those with a variety of other, undiagnosed conditions of infectious or endocrinologic etiology. The list of causes is extensive, and it is often necessary to rely on associated features of the presentation to suggest the direction of the workup (e.g., abdominal pain with acute intermittent porphyria or malar rash with systemic lupus erythematosus).
	Postictal psychosis is a syndrome that may follow a cluster of seizures (generalized or complex partial) in patients with long-standing epilepsy. Typically, the patient has a lucid interval lasting hours to days, followed by abrupt onset of psychosis. Psychotic symptoms include persecutory delusions, auditory hallucinations, and dysphoria. The episode usually resolves in days to weeks, but the psychosis can recur after subsequent seizure episodes, and with each recurrence it tends to lengthen in duration.
	Chronic interictal psychosis closely resembles psychosis in schizophrenia, with prominent delusions and auditory hallucinations. This syndrome is more common among patients with complex partial seizures, left temporal lobe foci, and/or medial temporal sclerosis on the left.
Laboratory testing	Particular demographics and presentation of the patient will determine which of the following laboratory evaluations should take precedence. For example, in a young male who appears "high," a urine toxicology screen may be an appropriate first step, whereas in an elderly woman taking levothyroxine, thyroid-stimulating hormone (TSH) may be indicated.
	• Comprehensive metabolic panel
	• Complete blood count with differential and platelets
	• TSH
	• Syphilis serology
	• HIV testing

Psychotic disorder due to another medical condition *(continued)*	
Laboratory testing *(continued)*	• Erythrocyte sedimentation rate or C-reactive protein • Blood alcohol level • Urine toxicology screen • Levels of prescribed drugs • Urinalysis • Head computed tomography (CT) with contrast or magnetic resonance imaging (MRI) with gadolinium • Electroencephalogram (EEG) • Electrocardiogram • Urine pregnancy testing • Lumbar puncture for cerebrospinal fluid analysis • Antinuclear antibody test • Cortisol (blood and 24-hour urine) • Spot urine for porphyrin precursors • Heavy metal screening • Vitamin B_{12} level • Ceruloplasmin and free serum copper levels • Antithyroid antibodies • Serum testosterone level • MRI with gadolinium (if CT done first)
	EEG in postictal psychosis is usually normal but may show mild generalized slowing. MRI may show medial temporal sclerosis or hippocampal atrophy that spares the anterior hippocampus.

American Psychiatric Association: Diagnostic and Statistical Manual of Mental Disorders, 5th Edition. Arlington, VA, American Psychiatric Association, 2013

Restless legs syndrome (RLS)	
Clinical diagnosis	RLS is characterized by an unpleasant sensation in the legs that gives rise to the urge to move that worsens during periods of rest or inactivity. The sensation is relieved by movement. The symptoms are most marked or are present exclusively during the evening or nighttime hours. The symptoms resemble those of akathisia. The nocturnal predominance results in significant sleep disruption. Periodic limb movements of sleep are often associated with RLS, but the two are distinct phenomena. RLS is also associated with panic disorder, generalized anxiety disorder, major depression, and fibromyalgia. It is more common in women than in men, and most patients present in middle age or older. It is associated with nighttime smoking.

In idiopathic RLS, the patient may report a positive family history of the condition. Secondary RLS most commonly occurs with iron deficiency anemia, in chronic conditions such as end-stage renal disease, or in pregnancy. Other associated conditions include chronic obstructive pulmonary disease, Parkinson's disease, stroke (in the basal ganglia, thalamus, or internal capsule), and diabetes. Whether the disease is primary or secondary, it may be exacerbated by antipsychotic and antidepressant medications (particularly selective serotonin reuptake inhibitors, serotonin-norepinephrine reuptake inhibitors, and mirtazapine). |
| Laboratory testing | Workup for iron deficiency anemia:

• Complete blood count with red cell indices

• Reticulocyte index

• Serum iron

• Total iron-binding capacity

• Ferritin

• Peripheral smear

Comprehensive metabolic panel |

Benes H, Walters AS, Allen RP, et al: Definition of restless legs syndrome, how to diagnose it, and how to differentiate it from RLS mimics. Mov Disord 22 (Suppl 18):S401–S408, 2007

Mohri I, Kato-Nishimura K, Tachibana N, et al: Restless legs syndrome (RLS): an unrecognized cause for bedtime problems and insomnia in children. Sleep Med 9(6):701–702, 2008

Sarcoidosis	
Clinical diagnosis	Sarcoidosis is a multisystem inflammatory disease involving granuloma formation, most commonly in the lungs, liver, skin, and eye. Nervous system involvement occurs in 5%–25% of patients. Presenting complaints are most often pulmonary, usually including cough and dyspnea. Skin lesions are nonspecific. Constitutional symptoms include fatigue, fever, night sweats, and weight loss. Nervous system lesions can occur anywhere in the brain, spinal cord, or peripheral nerves. Signs and symptoms include the following: • Transient CN VII paralysis (resembling Bell's palsy) • Blindness, visual changes • Hypothalamic/pituitary-driven endocrinological changes (hyperphagia, hyperprolactinemia, diabetes insipidus, hypothyroidism, hypogonadism, adrenocortical insufficiency) • Cognitive deficits of variable severity in about 50% (e.g., amnestic syndrome, dementia) • Personality change (with frontal lobe features) • Delirium • Seizures in about 15% • Hydrocephalus in about 5% • Peripheral neuropathy • Psychosis (rare) • Stroke (rare)
Laboratory testing	• Magnetic resonance imaging (MRI) may show hyperintensities on T2-weighted scans. • Basilar meningitis is the most common MRI finding. • MRI with gadolinium may show large, space-occupying masses on T1-weighted scans, or may be negative due to small size of the lesions or the effects of prior treatment with steroids. • Cerebrospinal fluid (CSF) may show lymphocytic pleocytosis with mildly increased protein, decreased glucose, increased immunoglobulin G index, and oligoclonal bands. Elevated levels of angiotensin-converting enzyme (ACE) are seen in CSF in about half of patients.

Sarcoidosis *(continued)*	
Laboratory testing *(continued)*	• Elevated levels of serum ACE (SACE) are seen in serum in two-thirds of patients with acute disease, but only one-fifth of those with chronic disease. Current use of an ACE inhibitor will cause a falsely low level. • The diagnosis is confirmed by tissue biopsy of an affected organ, usually the lung.

Costabel U, Ohshimo S, Guzman J: Diagnosis of sarcoidosis. Curr Opin Pulm Med 14(5):455–461, 2008

Fauci AS, Braunwald E, Kasper DL, et al (eds): Harrison's Principles of Internal Medicine, 17th Edition. New York, McGraw-Hill, 2008

Judson MA: The diagnosis of sarcoidosis. Clin Chest Med 29(3):415–427, viii, 2008

Parrish S, Turner JF: Diagnosis of sarcoidosis. Dis Mon 55(11):693–703, 2009

Schizophrenia	
Clinical diagnosis	Schizophrenia is characterized by two or more of the following symptoms, each present for a significant portion of time during a 1-month period (less if treated): delusions, hallucinations, disorganized speech, grossly disorganized or catatonic behavior, or negative symptoms (restricted affect, avolition). At least one symptom should be from the first three listed. Function at work, interpersonal relations, or self-care is impaired. Continuous signs of the disturbance persist for at least 6 months.

The diagnosis is excluded when there is evidence for schizoaffective disorder or a mood disorder with psychotic features, or when the disturbance is due to the effects of a drug or another medical condition. If there is a history of autism spectrum disorder or a communication disorder of childhood onset, the additional diagnosis of schizophrenia is made only if prominent delusions or hallucinations and other required symptoms of schizophrenia are also present for at least 1 month (less if treated). |
| Laboratory testing | For the patient presenting with acute psychosis, a laboratory investigation directed toward the exclusion of potential medical causes or contributors is indicated. The choice of test(s) will be determined by specific symptoms and patient demographics.

Tests to be considered include the following:

• Comprehensive metabolic panel

• Complete blood count with differential and platelets

• Thyroid-stimulating hormone (TSH)

• Syphilis serology

• HIV testing

• Erythrocyte sedimentation rate or C-reactive protein

• Blood alcohol level

• Urine toxicology screen

• Levels of prescribed drugs

• Urinalysis

• Head computed tomography (CT) with contrast or magnetic resonance imaging (MRI) with gadolinium

• Electroencephalogram

• Electrocardiogram

• Urine pregnancy testing

• Lumbar puncture for cerebrospinal fluid analysis

• Antinuclear antibody test |

Schizophrenia *(continued)*	
Laboratory testing *(continued)*	• Cortisol (blood and 24-hour urine) • Spot urine for porphyrin precursors • Heavy metal screening • Vitamin B_{12} level • Ceruloplasmin and free serum copper levels • Antithyroid antibodies • Serum testosterone level • MRI with gadolinium (if CT done first) Patients with schizophrenia who are being treated with antipsychotic medications will require monitoring lab tests ("safety labs") as outlined in Chapter 3, "Psychotropic Medications." In addition, vigilance in monitoring for tardive dyskinesia (for conventional antipsychotics) and metabolic syndrome (for atypical antipsychotics) will be required. Laboratory tests used to diagnose the metabolic syndrome are covered under that entry. Depending on the patient's exposure history, HIV and/or tuberculosis testing may also be indicated.

American Psychiatric Association: Diagnostic and Statistical Manual of Mental Disorders, 5th Edition. Arlington, VA, American Psychiatric Association, 2013

Syndrome of inappropriate antidiuretic hormone secretion (SIADH)

Clinical diagnosis	Patients at risk of SIADH (see Figure 5 in the Appendix) include the elderly, particularly those resident in nursing homes, as well as those with the following conditions: • Central nervous system disease—infection (meningitis, encephalitis, abscess, Rocky Mountain spotted fever, AIDS), stroke, traumatic brain injury, brain tumor, hydrocephalus, subdural hematoma, subarachnoid hemorrhage, cavernous sinus thrombosis, delirium tremens, acute intermittent porphyria, multiple sclerosis, Guillain-Barré syndrome, Shy-Drager syndrome • Cancer—lung, oropharynx, gastrointestinal tract, genitourinary tract; lymphomas, sarcomas • Pulmonary disease—infection (including viral and bacterial pneumonia, abscess, tuberculosis), asthma, cystic fibrosis, respiratory failure • Use of certain drugs—including selective serotonin reuptake inhibitors, tricyclic antidepressants, carbamazepine, nicotine, opioids, antipsychotics, nonsteroidal anti-inflammatory drugs, and 3,4-methylenedioxymethamphetamine (MDMA; Ecstasy) • Transient conditions—general anesthesia, pain, nausea, stress, endurance exercise Rapid development of severe hyponatremia in SIADH (serum sodium <125 mEq/L) may be associated with the following severe signs and symptoms: • Confusion • Hallucinations • Delirium • Seizures • Coma • Decerebrate posture • Respiratory arrest This syndrome can be fatal.

Syndrome of inappropriate antidiuretic hormone secretion (SIADH) *(continued)*

Clinical diagnosis *(continued)*	Milder sodium reductions may be associated with the following: • Headache • Difficulty concentrating • Memory impairment • Weakness • Muscle cramps • Dysgeusia Chronic hyponatremia may be asymptomatic, although affected patients may have subtle neurological deficits that lead to falls.
Laboratory testing	Check serum and urine osmolality, serum and urine sodium, and blood urea nitrogen (BUN). SIADH is diagnosed when the following criteria are met: • Decreased effective osmolality (<275 mOsm/kg); effective osmolality = measured osmolality minus the value of BUN/2.8, where BUN is measured in mg/dL • Urine osmolality >100 mOsm/kg • Clinical euvolemia (absence of orthostasis, tachycardia, decreased skin turgor, dry mucous membranes, edema, and ascites) • Urinary sodium >40 mEq/L with normal salt intake in diet • Normal thyroid and adrenal function • No recent use of diuretics Note that hyponatremia is not included in the diagnostic criteria, although symptoms do not appear unless sodium is low, and sodium level is usually <130 mEq/L.

Ellison DH, Berl T: Clinical practice. The syndrome of inappropriate antidiuresis. N Engl J Med 356(20):2064–2072, 2007

Fauci AS, Braunwald E, Kasper DL, et al (eds): Harrison's Principles of Internal Medicine, 17th Edition. New York, McGraw-Hill, 2008

Kasper DL, Fauci AS, Hauser SL, et al (eds): Harrison's Principles of Internal Medicine, 19th Edition. New York, McGraw-Hill, 2015

Robinson AG: Disorders of antidiuretic hormone secretion. Clin Endocrinol Metab 14(1):55–88, 1985

Thiamine (vitamin B₁) deficiency	
Clinical diagnosis	Patients at risk of thiamine deficiency include the elderly; postsurgical patients (gastric bypass or other gastrointestinal surgeries); patients with alcoholism, eating disorders (anorexia or bulimia), chronic diarrhea (e.g., lithium-induced), chronic vomiting (e.g., pyloric stenosis, hyperemesis gravidarum), AIDS, thyrotoxicosis, or Crohn's disease; patients treated with diuretics for chronic heart failure; and patients treated with chemotherapeutic agents for cancer. It is likely that several genetic defects contribute to development of the symptoms of clinical deficiency in the presence of one of these conditions. Two classic syndromes are recognized: cardiovascular (wet beriberi) and neurological (dry beriberi). Certain population associations have been noted: Asians tend to develop cardiovascular syndromes, and Europeans tend to develop neurological syndromes. Cardiovascular and neurological syndromes may coexist. Cardiac signs (heart failure, usually high-output): • Tachycardia • S_3 • Apical systolic murmur • Widened pulse pressure (systolic blood pressure minus diastolic blood pressure) • Elevated ventricular filling pressures • Electrocardiogram: decreased voltage, prolonged QT, T-wave abnormalities • Chest X ray: cardiomegaly, pulmonary congestion • Peripheral edema Neurological signs: • Severe, short-term thiamine deficiency induces Wernicke encephalopathy, whereas mild to moderate, long-term deficiency induces a peripheral neuropathy. • The classic clinical triad of Wernicke encephalopathy—confusion, ataxia, and ophthalmoplegia—is seen in less than 20% of cases. Most cases present as an isolated delirium. Ophthalmoplegic signs range from nystagmus to complete inability to abduct the eyes (CN VI palsy). • Korsakoff syndrome usually develops as a chronic condition after repeated episodes of Wernicke encephalopathy, but it can develop with the first episode. Korsakoff syndrome is manifested as amnesia, which is usually marked, with confabulation variably present.

Thiamine (vitamin B$_1$) deficiency *(continued)*	
Clinical diagnosis *(continued)*	Neurological signs *(continued)*: • Peripheral neuropathy manifests as acute or subacute onset of paresthesias, dysesthesias, and mild lower-extremity weakness; signs include stocking-glove sensory loss, distal leg and foot weakness, and absent ankle jerks. Neuropathy is worse distally than proximally and involves myelin more than axons. • The spectrum of neurological signs and symptoms includes nonspecific mental status changes such as apathy, low energy, fatigue, slowness, memory and other cognitive impairments, and disturbance of consciousness ranging from inattention to coma. *Confusion* is the term most commonly applied, although some patients also have hallucinations, delusions, and behavioral disturbances and are diagnosed with delirium.
Laboratory testing	Thiamine levels consistent with deficiency: • Whole blood <275 ng/g hemoglobin (Hb) (<0.65 nmol/g Hb) • Red blood cell (thiamine pyrophosphate) <4.5 µg/dL (<106 nmol/L)

Mulholland PJ: Susceptibility of the cerebellum to thiamine deficiency. Cerebellum 5(11):55–63, 2006

O'Keeffe ST: Thiamine deficiency in elderly people. Age Ageing 29(2):99–101, 2000

Rao SN, Chandak GR: Cardiac beriberi: often a missed diagnosis. J Trop Pediatr 56(4):284–285, 2010

Sechi G, Serra A: Wernicke's encephalopathy: new clinical settings and recent advances in diagnosis and management. Lancet Neurol 6(5):442–455, 2007

Tuberculosis (TB)	
Clinical diagnosis	TB is a bacterial infection caused by the acid-fast bacillus *Mycobacterium tuberculosis*, which primarily affects the pulmonary system but can involve many other organ systems, including the brain and meninges. It is spread by airborne droplets from infected persons through coughing, sneezing, or breathing. Patients at risk include residents of correctional facilities, chronic mental health facilities, and nursing homes. At even higher risk are those who are homeless and those with alcoholism, intravenous drug abuse, HIV/AIDS, or chronic liver or kidney disease. Most people who are infected develop latent TB, in which the bacteria are limited to a few cells and remain inactive. These patients are asymptomatic and noninfectious, but about 10% of those who go untreated will later develop active TB. Patients who become immunocompromised can also develop active TB, with symptoms dependent on the organ system affected. Patients with active pulmonary TB exhibit cough (sometimes with bloody sputum), fever, chills, weakness, and weight loss. Those with spinal TB exhibit back pain and paralysis. Other sites of infection include joints, bone marrow, urinary system, reproductive system, and heart. Miliary TB involves infection of the blood itself and can result in multiple TB emboli. In the central nervous system, TB typically involves the meninges, where it causes basilar meningitis, or the brain parenchyma, where it causes masses known as tuberculomas. • Meningitis causes delirium, stiff neck, fever, and headache. The syndrome of inappropriate antidiuretic hormone secretion (SIADH) can be seen, as can III, IV, and VI cranial nerve palsies. Less commonly, obstructive hydrocephalus is seen. Other sequelae include basal ganglia infarctions with tremor, chorea, and dystonia. • Inflammation of both large pial and small penetrating arteries can occur, with consequent territorial or lacunar infarctions. • With tuberculomas, symptoms depend on the brain area affected; these masses are usually multiple and can be supratentorial or infratentorial. Seizures can occur.
Laboratory testing	• Latent TB can be diagnosed by a positive purified protein derivative (PPD) skin test. • In patients with TB meningitis and tuberculomas, the PPD skin test is usually positive. • False-negative PPD tests are common in AIDS patients. • Meningitis and tuberculomas may be visualized on contrast-enhanced computed tomography or magnetic resonance imaging.

Tuberculosis (TB) *(continued)*	
Laboratory testing *(continued)*	• Cerebrospinal fluid (CSF) in meningitis shows a pleocytosis (initially polymorphonuclear leukocytes; later lymphocytes), low blood sugar, and elevated protein. Smears usually yield no results. CSF cultures are positive in three-quarters of patients but may take weeks to return.
	• Polymerase chain reaction (PCR) allows rapid detection of TB in cases of meningitis.
	• In tuberculomas, CSF is normal or only mildly abnormal.

Brodie D, Schluger NW: The diagnosis of tuberculosis. Clin Chest Med 26:247–271, vi, 2005

Cain KP, McCarthy KD, Heilig CM, et al: An algorithm for tuberculosis screening and diagnosis in people with HIV. N Engl J Med 362(8):707–716, 2010

Phypers M, Harris T, Power C: CNS tuberculosis: a longitudinal analysis of epidemiological and clinical features. Int J Tuberc Lung Dis 10(1):99–103, 2006

Vitamin B$_{12}$ deficiency	
Clinical diagnosis	Patients at risk of vitamin B$_{12}$ (cyanocobalamin) deficiency include the elderly, those who are malnourished (e.g., with anorexia nervosa), strict vegetarians, patients who have undergone gastric or ileal resection, and those with malabsorption syndromes. Among the elderly, the most common type of B$_{12}$ deficiency is pernicious anemia, which is caused by deficiency of intrinsic factor due to chronic atrophic gastritis.

Although the deficiency may develop very slowly, once B$_{12}$ stores have reached a critical threshold, symptoms become apparent over weeks to months. More acute onset can be seen in marginally deficient patients administered nitrous oxide as a dental anesthetic.

The degenerative process of B$_{12}$ deficiency involves demyelination within the brain and spinal cord and in peripheral nerves, with eventual axonal loss if untreated. Brain involvement can occur without spinal cord involvement or anemia.

Cerebral signs and symptoms of B$_{12}$ deficiency include the following:

• Chronic cognitive impairment (dementia)

• Confusion and/or delirium

• Depression

• Personality change

• Mania

• Psychosis ("megaloblastic madness")

Spinal cord and peripheral nerves are affected in tandem. In the spinal cord, the classic syndrome of subacute combined degeneration involves demyelination in posterior columns and lateral corticospinal tracts. Corticospinal degeneration is most evident in the lower cord and posterior column degeneration in the upper cord. Signs and symptoms include the following:

• Paresthesias

• Numbness

• Distal weakness

• Loss of vibration sense

• Loss of light touch, pinprick, and position sense

• Ataxia

• Positive Romberg sign

• Extensor plantar responses

• Hyperreflexia or hyporeflexia

• Spasticity of lower extremities

• Incontinence |

Vitamin B$_{12}$ deficiency *(continued)*	
Laboratory testing	Macrocytic anemia is variably present. The blood smear may show hypersegmented neutrophils and macro-ovalocytes. Cerebral involvement can occur without cord or peripheral nerve involvement and without anemia or macrocytosis. In elderly patients, given the high pretest probability of deficiency in the presence of characteristic symptoms, it is a common practice to replace B$_{12}$ for any patient with a B$_{12}$ level <400 pg/mL. Methylmalonic acid and homocysteine levels are more sensitive indicators of B$_{12}$ deficiency, as both increase in the deficient state. These labs also provide the means to distinguish folate deficiency. In folate deficiency, the homocysteine level is high, but the methylmalonic acid level is normal. A newer metabolic marker, the cobalamin transporter holotranscobalamin (holoTC), can also be measured in serum. This marker is in fact a better measure of cobalamin deficiency than the B$_{12}$ level itself because it assays only the active part of the molecule. The reference range for holoTC is 19–134 pmol/L. This test is not yet clinically available. In the workup of pernicious anemia, the Schilling test has generally fallen out of use in favor of anti–parietal cell and anti–intrinsic factor antibody levels. If these are normal, then other causes of B$_{12}$ deficiency are considered. Complete blood count (CBC) may show macrocytic anemia, or only macrocytosis (elevated mean corpuscular volume [MCV]). In one-third of cases with brain involvement (e.g., cognitive impairment or depression), no macrocytosis is seen. Magnetic resonance imaging may show patchy hyperintensities on T2-weighted images in the centrum semiovale, more prominent in frontal lobes. Electroencephalogram may show generalized slowing or slowing of the posterior dominant frequency. Cerebrospinal fluid is usually unremarkable except for slightly increased protein. To monitor the effectiveness of vitamin B$_{12}$ replacement: • Perform CBC after 2 weeks to document increase in hemoglobin and decrease in MCV. • Perform CBC after 8 weeks to document resolution of anemia. • B$_{12}$ level does not need to be checked unless noncompliance is suspected with oral therapy.

Hvas AM, Nexo E: Diagnosis and treatment of vitamin B$_{12}$ deficiency: an update. Haematologica 91(11):1506–1512, 2006

Kim JM, Stewart R, Kim SW, et al: Predictive value of folate, vitamin B$_{12}$ and homocysteine levels in late-life depression. Br J Psychiatry 192(4):268–274, 2008

Lerner V, Kanevsky M, Dwolatzky T, et al: Vitamin B$_{12}$ and folate serum levels in newly admitted psychiatric patients. Clin Nutr 25(1):60–67, 2006

Wernicke-Korsakoff syndrome	
Clinical diagnosis	*Wernicke encephalopathy*
	• This condition usually occurs in patients with alcoholism but can affect other thiamine-deficient patients, such as those with anorexia nervosa.
	• Onset is usually subacute, but it can be acute if glucose load is given before thiamine in a marginally thiamine-deficient patient.
	• The classic triad is mental status changes (delirium), ataxia, and ophthalmoplegia (often just nystagmus).
	• The fully developed triad is actually seen in <20% of cases.
	• The patient may simply "look drunk."
	• In untreated patients, nystagmus progresses to a CN VI palsy, in which the patient is unable to abduct the eyes, and in some cases to complete ophthalmoplegia.
	• Seizures can occur.
	• Vital signs are often abnormal: hypothermia, tachycardia, and postural hypotension can be seen.
	• Death may ensue.
	• Those who survive are often left with some residual deficit, most often the dense amnesia of Korsakoff syndrome.
	Korsakoff syndrome (Korsakoff psychosis)
	• Approximately 80% of patients with Wernicke encephalopathy who survive develop Korsakoff syndrome.
	• Often undiagnosed in life, even when clear pathological findings are seen at autopsy.
	• Characterized by severe anterograde amnesia.
	• Some degree of retrograde amnesia may be seen, with a temporal gradient.
	• Many patients have a tendency to confabulate.
	• Patients are often indifferent to symptoms.
	• Some degree of ophthalmoplegia and ataxia, which are sequelae of Wernicke encephalopathy, can be seen.

Wernicke-Korsakoff syndrome *(continued)*

Laboratory testing	A thiamine level can be drawn, but in the setting of Wernicke encephalopathy the result usually takes too long to be useful. This condition is a medically urgent one and requires immediate treatment with parenteral thiamine. Magnetic resonance imaging (MRI) can assist in confirming the diagnosis after acute treatment has commenced: • MRI is used to rule out Wernicke encephalopathy (low sensitivity, high specificity). • Coronal sections through the mammillary bodies should be requested, with a clinical note *"to evaluate Wernicke-Korsakoff syndrome."* • In Wernicke encephalopathy, abnormal signal intensity is seen in the mammillary bodies on diffusion-weighted imaging, fluid-attenuated inversion recovery (FLAIR), and T2-weighted scans. • In Korsakoff syndrome, T2-weighted scans show atrophy of the mammillary bodies. • Other brain areas that may be affected in Wernicke-Korsakoff syndrome include periaqueductal gray, midbrain tectum, dorsomedial nucleus of the thalamus, and mammillothalamic tract.

Descombes E, Dessibourg CA, Fellay G: Acute encephalopathy due to thiamine deficiency (Wernicke's encephalopathy) in a chronic hemodialyzed patient: a case report. Clin Nephrol 35(4):171–175, 1991

Sechi G, Serra A: Wernicke's encephalopathy: new clinical settings and recent advances in diagnosis and management. Lancet Neurol 6(5):442–455, 2007

CHAPTER 3

Psychotropic Medications

Laboratory Screening and Monitoring

Acamprosate (Campral)	
Screening laboratory tests	• Blood urea nitrogen (BUN), creatinine, and estimated glomerular filtration rate (GFR) • Pregnancy test in women who could become pregnant
Monitoring laboratory tests	• Periodic monitoring of BUN, creatinine, and estimated GFR • Electrocardiogram if signs/symptoms such as palpitations, angina, or syncope develop

American Society of Health-System Pharmacists: AHFS Drug Information 2016. Bethesda, MD, American Society of Health-System Pharmacists, 2016

Package Insert. National Library of Medicine DailyMed. Available at: https://dailymed.nlm.nih.gov. Accessed May 2016.

Amphetamines (Adderall); dextroamphetamines (Dexedrine); lisdexamfetamine dimesylate (Vyvanse)	
Screening laboratory tests	• Electrocardiogram (ECG) and echocardiogram in patients with family history of sudden death or ventricular arrhythmias or with physical findings suggestive of cardiovascular disease • Thyroid-stimulating hormone (TSH) • Fasting blood glucose • Pregnancy test in women who could become pregnant • Consider electroencephalogram (EEG) in patients with a history suggestive of seizure disorder.
Monitoring laboratory tests	• Prompt cardiac evaluation (ECG, echocardiogram) if syncope, exertional chest pain, or other cardiovascular symptoms develop • EEG if signs/symptoms of seizure develop • Periodic check of blood glucose and TSH • Growth rate (height) and weight measurements for children

American Society of Health-System Pharmacists: AHFS Drug Information 2016. Bethesda, MD, American Society of Health-System Pharmacists, 2016

Package Inserts. National Library of Medicine DailyMed. Available at: https://dailymed.nlm. nih.gov. Accessed May 2016.

Antipsychotic medications, first-generation (typical)*	
Screening laboratory tests	• Fasting glucose (or hemoglobin A_{1C}) • Fasting lipid profile • Complete blood count (CBC) with differential • Blood chemistries: electrolytes, renal function, liver function, thyroid function • Electrocardiogram (ECG) • Abnormal Involuntary Movement Scale (AIMS) assessment—baseline • Pregnancy test in women who could become pregnant
Monitoring laboratory tests	• Fasting glucose (or hemoglobin A_{1C}) and lipid profile every 6 months • Periodic check of CBC with differential for patients taking phenothiazines • Blood chemistries: electrolytes, renal function, liver function, thyroid function annually and as clinically indicated • Prolactin level check for symptoms of hyperprolactinemia • ECG for any cardiac symptoms • ECG every 6 months for patients taking thioridazine, mesoridazine, or pimozide • AIMS assessment every 6 months (every 3 months in elderly patients)

*Includes chlorpromazine, haloperidol, perphenazine, thioridazine, and others.

American Psychiatric Association: Practice guideline for the treatment of patients with schizophrenia, second edition. Am J Psychiatry 161(2, Suppl):1–56, 2004

American Society of Health-System Pharmacists: AHFS Drug Information 2016. Bethesda, MD, American Society of Health-System Pharmacists, 2016

Antipsychotic medications, second-generation (atypical)*	
Screening laboratory tests	• Fasting glucose (or hemoglobin A_{1C}) • Fasting lipid profile • Electrocardiogram (ECG) • Complete blood count (CBC) with differential • Blood chemistries: electrolytes, renal function, liver function, thyroid function (thyroid-stimulating hormone) • Pregnancy test in women who could become pregnant *Physical measurements:* • Weight, height, body mass index (BMI) calculation, and waist circumference • Blood pressure and pulse (sitting and standing), temperature • Abnormal Involuntary Movement Scale (AIMS) assessment—baseline
Monitoring laboratory tests	• Weight and BMI calculation at 4 weeks, 8 weeks, 12 weeks, and then quarterly • Waist circumference yearly • Blood pressure, pulse, and temperature at 12 weeks and then yearly • Fasting glucose (or hemoglobin A_{1C}) at 12 weeks and then yearly • Fasting lipid profile at 12 weeks and then every 5 years • Periodic check of CBC for patients taking clozapine, olanzapine, brexiprazole, or cariprazine • Blood chemistries: electrolytes, renal function, liver function, thyroid function annually and as clinically indicated • ECG every 6 months for patients taking ziprasidone; yearly for all others • Prolactin level check for symptoms of hyperprolactinemia • AIMS assessment every 12 months (every 6 months for elderly patients)

*Includes aripiprazole, asenapine, brexiprazole, cariprazine, iloperidone, lurasidone, olanzapine, paliperidone, quetiapine, risperidone, and ziprasidone. Clozapine is covered separately.

American Society of Health-System Pharmacists: AHFS Drug Information 2016. Bethesda, MD, American Society of Health-System Pharmacists, 2016

Olufadi R, Byrne CD: Clinical and laboratory diagnosis of the metabolic syndrome. J Clin Pathol 61(6):697–706, 2008

Otsuka: Brexiprazole (package insert). Available at: https://www.otsuka-us.com/media/static/Rexulti-PI.pdf. Accessed June 10, 2016.

Package Inserts. National Library of Medicine DailyMed. Available at: https://dailymed.nlm. nih.gov. Accessed June 2016.

Atomoxetine (Strattera)	
Screening laboratory tests	• Electrocardiogram (ECG) and echocardiogram in patients with family history of sudden death or ventricular arrhythmias, or with physical findings suggestive of cardiovascular disease • Liver function tests (LFTs) to determine whether dosage adjustment is needed • Pregnancy test in women who could become pregnant
Monitoring laboratory tests	• Prompt cardiac evaluation (ECG, echocardiogram) if syncope, exertional chest pain, or other cardiovascular symptoms develop • LFTs with first signs of hepatic dysfunction (jaundice, dark urine, pruritis, right upper quadrant tenderness, or flu-like symptoms). Drug should be discontinued and not reinstated in patients with jaundice or laboratory evidence of hepatic injury. • Growth rate (height) and weight measurements for children

American Society of Health-System Pharmacists: AHFS Drug Information 2016. Bethesda, MD, American Society of Health-System Pharmacists, 2016

Package Insert. National Library of Medicine DailyMed. Available at: https://dailymed.nlm. nih.gov. Accessed May 2016.

Benzodiazepines*	
Screening laboratory tests	When a benzodiazepine is considered for the treatment of anxiety, liver function tests may be indicated, depending on the particular drug to be used. In patients with liver impairment, dosage adjustment may be necessary, especially with long-acting benzodiazepines. Height and weight measurements to calculate the baseline body mass index, as indicated.
Monitoring laboratory tests	No specific laboratory monitoring is indicated for benzodiazepines per se, although the metabolism of certain drugs may be affected by hepatic or renal dysfunction, aging, or the development of obesity. Drug level testing may be indicated in selected cases. (See individual drug level entries in Chapter 1, "Laboratory Tests," for details.)

*Includes alprazolam, chlordiazepoxide, clonazepam, diazepam, lorazepam, oxazepam, and temazepam.

American Society of Health-System Pharmacists: AHFS Drug Information 2016. Bethesda, MD, American Society of Health-System Pharmacists, 2016

Package Inserts. National Library of Medicine DailyMed. Available at: https://dailymed.nlm.nih.gov. Accessed May 2016.

Buprenorphine (Buprenex, Subutex); **buprenorphine/naloxone (Suboxone)**	
Screening laboratory tests	• Liver function panel, including gamma-glutamyltransferase (GGT)
	• Hepatitis B and C screening
	• Thyroid-stimulating hormone; free thyroxine (T_4), triiodothyronine (T_3) if indicated
	• Pregnancy test in women who could become pregnant
Monitoring laboratory tests	• Periodic check of liver functioning, including GGT
	• Urine drug screening

American Society of Health-System Pharmacists: AHFS Drug Information 2016. Bethesda, MD, American Society of Health-System Pharmacists, 2016

Package Inserts. U.S. National Library of Medicine DailyMed. Available at: https://dailymed.nlm.nih.gov. Accessed May 2016.

Bupropion (Aplenzin, Budeprion SR, Wellbutrin)	
Screening laboratory tests	• Liver function panel • Blood urea nitrogen (BUN), creatinine, and estimation of glomerular filtration rate (GFR) • Pregnancy test in women who could become pregnant
Monitoring laboratory tests	• Liver function panel, BUN, creatinine, and estimation of GFR every 6–12 months • Electrocardiogram for palpitations or other cardiovascular signs/ symptoms • Electroencephalogram for signs/symptoms suggestive of seizure

American Society of Health-System Pharmacists: AHFS Drug Information 2016. Bethesda, MD, American Society of Health-System Pharmacists, 2016

Package Inserts. National Library of Medicine DailyMed. Available at: https://dailymed.nlm. nih.gov. Accessed May 2016.

Buspirone	
Screening laboratory tests	Although buspirone is hepatically metabolized, its level is affected only by significant liver disease such as cirrhosis. No specific laboratory tests are recommended for the initiation of buspirone.
Monitoring laboratory tests	No specific laboratory tests are recommended to monitor buspirone treatment.

American Society of Health-System Pharmacists: AHFS Drug Information 2016. Bethesda, MD, American Society of Health-System Pharmacists, 2016

Package Insert. National Library of Medicine DailyMed. Available at: https://dailymed.nlm. nih.gov. Accessed May 2016.

Carbamazepine	
Screening laboratory tests	• Electrolytes • Blood urea nitrogen (BUN) and creatinine • Liver function tests (LFTs), including aspartate transaminase (AST), alanine transaminase (ALT), bilirubin, alkaline phosphatase (ALP), and lactate dehydrogenase (LDH) • Complete blood count (CBC) with differential and platelets • Thyroid-stimulating hormone (TSH) • Pregnancy test in women who could become pregnant *Metabolic syndrome screening* • Fasting glucose (or hemoglobin A_{1C}) • Fasting lipid profile • Weight, height, body mass index (BMI) calculation, and waist circumference • Blood pressure
Monitoring laboratory tests	• CBC with platelets, electrolytes, and LFTs should be checked every 2 weeks for the first 2 months of treatment. • Thereafter, periodic checks should be made of CBC with platelets, LFTs, BUN, creatinine, electrolytes (especially serum sodium for hyponatremia with carbamazepine during the first 3 months), and TSH. • If carbamazepine levels are drawn, these should be trough levels taken just before the morning dose of medication. • Levels should be drawn 5 days after initiation of therapy or any change in dose. *Metabolic syndrome monitoring* • Weight and BMI calculation at 4 weeks, 8 weeks, 12 weeks, and then quarterly • Waist circumference yearly • Blood pressure at 12 weeks and then yearly • Fasting glucose (or hemoglobin A_{1C}) at 12 weeks and then yearly • Fasting lipid profile at 12 weeks and then every 5 years

Hirschfeld RMA, Bowden CL, Gitlin MJ, et al; Work Group on Bipolar Disorder: Practice Guideline for the Treatment of Patients With Bipolar Disorder, Second Edition. Washington, DC, American Psychiatric Association, 2002. Available at: http://psychiatryonline.org/pb/assets/raw/sitewide/practice_guidelines/guidelines/bipolar.pdf. Accessed May 2016; Guideline watch: http://psychiatryonline.org/pb/assets/raw/sitewide/practice_guidelines/guidelines/bipolar-watch.pdf.
Olufadi R, Byrne CD: Clinical and laboratory diagnosis of the metabolic syndrome. J Clin Pathol 61(6):697–706, 2008

Clozapine (Clozaril, FazaClo, Versacloz)	
Screening laboratory tests	Clinicians who prescribe clozapine are now required to register and demonstrate competence in its prescription. See the Web site https://www.clozapinerems.com. • Complete blood count that includes an absolute neutrophil count (ANC). *To be eligible for clozapine, the patient must have an ANC ≥1,500/mm³ (1,500/μL) or ≥1,000/mm³ in those with documented benign ethnic neutropenia.* • Electrocardiogram (ECG) • Sedimentation rate or C-reactive protein • Drug levels for patients taking anticonvulsant drugs (to ensure therapeutic range) • Pregnancy test in women who could become pregnant *Metabolic syndrome screening* • Fasting blood glucose (or hemoglobin A_{1C}) • Fasting lipid profile, including triglycerides • Weight, height, body mass index (BMI) calculation, and waist circumference • Blood pressure (including orthostatic)
Monitoring laboratory tests	*Hematologic (ANC) monitoring frequency* • Weekly from initiation to 6 months • Every 2 weeks from 6–12 months • Monthly after 12 months • For hospice patients: every 6 months • If neutropenia develops, its severity determines what actions to take. See https://www.clozapinerems.com. *Monitoring for cardiovascular effects* • Eosinophil count weekly for the first month • Sedimentation rate or C-reactive protein weekly for the first month • Troponins weekly for the first month • ECG annually

Clozapine (Clozaril, FazaClo, Versacloz) *(continued)*	
Monitoring laboratory tests *(continued)*	*Metabolic syndrome monitoring* • Fasting blood glucose monthly at the beginning of treatment, then annually • Lipid profile at 3 months and annually • Weight, BMI calculation, and waist circumference at 3 months and annually • Blood pressure (including orthostatic) daily for the first 2 weeks of treatment, at each dose escalation, and annually as a routine

American Society of Health-System Pharmacists: AHFS Drug Information 2016. Bethesda, MD, American Society of Health-System Pharmacists, 2016

Package Inserts. National Library of Medicine DailyMed. Available at: https://dailymed.nlm. nih.gov. Accessed May 2016.

Donepezil (Aricept)	
Screening laboratory tests	• Although no specific laboratory screening is recommended by the manufacturer, an electrocardiogram may be considered to exclude supraventricular conduction abnormalities before initiating treatment. • Pregnancy test in women who could become pregnant
Monitoring laboratory tests	No specific laboratory monitoring is recommended by the manufacturer.

American Society of Health-System Pharmacists: AHFS Drug Information 2016. Bethesda, MD, American Society of Health-System Pharmacists, 2016

Package Insert. National Library of Medicine DailyMed. Available at: https://dailymed.nlm. nih.gov. Accessed May 2016.

Duloxetine (Cymbalta)	
Screening laboratory tests	• No specific laboratory testing is recommended by the manufacturer. • Consider liver function tests (LFTs), including aspartate transaminase (AST), alanine transaminase (ALT), alkaline phosphatase (ALP), and bilirubin. • Consider baseline serum sodium. • Pregnancy test in women who could become pregnant
Monitoring laboratory tests	• LFTs monthly for the first 3 months of treatment, then every 6 months • Electrolytes to check sodium level if patient develops symptoms of syndrome of inappropriate antidiuretic hormone secretion (SIADH)

American Society of Health-System Pharmacists: AHFS Drug Information 2016. Bethesda, MD, American Society of Health-System Pharmacists, 2016

Package Insert. National Library of Medicine DailyMed. Available at: https://dailymed.nlm. nih.gov. Accessed May 2016.

Gabapentin	
Screening laboratory tests	• Blood urea nitrogen and creatinine, with estimation of glomerular filtration rate • Pregnancy test in women who could become pregnant
Monitoring laboratory tests	• No specific laboratory monitoring is recommended.

American Society of Health-System Pharmacists: AHFS Drug Information 2016. Bethesda, MD, American Society of Health-System Pharmacists, 2016

Package Insert. National Library of Medicine DailyMed. Available at: https://dailymed.nlm. nih.gov. Accessed May 2016.

Galantamine (Razadyne)	
Screening laboratory tests	• Although no specific laboratory testing is recommended by the manufacturer, a screening electrocardiogram (ECG) may be considered to exclude supraventricular conduction abnormalities before initiating treatment. • Blood urea nitrogen (BUN), creatinine, and liver function tests (LFTs) should be performed to determine whether dosage adjustment is needed. • Pregnancy test in women who could become pregnant
Monitoring laboratory tests	• Periodic check of ECG, BUN, creatinine, and LFTs

American Society of Health-System Pharmacists: AHFS Drug Information 2016. Bethesda, MD, American Society of Health-System Pharmacists, 2016

Package Insert. National Library of Medicine DailyMed. Available at: https://dailymed.nlm. nih.gov. Accessed May 2016.

Lamotrigine (Lamictal)	
Screening laboratory tests	• Blood urea nitrogen (BUN), creatinine, and estimation of glomerular filtration rate • Liver function tests (LFTs) • Pregnancy test in women who could become pregnant
Monitoring laboratory tests	• Periodic check of BUN, creatinine, and LFTs

American Society of Health-System Pharmacists: AHFS Drug Information 2016. Bethesda, MD, American Society of Health-System Pharmacists, 2016

Package Insert. National Library of Medicine DailyMed. Available at: https://dailymed.nlm. nih.gov. Accessed May 2016.

Levetiracetam (Keppra)	
Screening laboratory tests	• Blood urea nitrogen, creatinine, and estimated glomerular filtration rate • Pregnancy test in women who could become pregnant
Monitoring laboratory tests	• Periodic check of complete blood count with differential and liver function tests, as indicated by clinical findings

American Society of Health-System Pharmacists: AHFS Drug Information 2016. Bethesda, MD, American Society of Health-System Pharmacists, 2016

Package Insert. National Library of Medicine DailyMed. Available at: https://dailymed.nlm. nih.gov. Accessed May 2016.

Lithium	
Screening laboratory tests	• Blood urea nitrogen (BUN), creatinine, and estimated glomerular filtration rate (GFR) • Complete blood count • Thyroid-stimulating hormone (TSH) • Electrocardiogram for patients >40 years and for any patient with preexisting cardiovascular disease • Pregnancy test in women who could become pregnant *Consider metabolic syndrome screening* • Fasting glucose (or hemoglobin A_{1C}) • Fasting lipid profile • Weight, height, body mass index (BMI) calculation, and waist circumference • Blood pressure
Monitoring laboratory tests	• Lithium level within 1 week of initiation (or change in dose) of drug, then every 2–3 months for the first 6 months of treatment. When lithium level is checked, blood is drawn 12 hours after the last dose (trough level). • BUN, creatinine, and estimated GFR every 2–3 months for the first 6 months • TSH check once or twice during the first 6 months • After 6 months, lithium level, BUN, creatinine, and TSH every 6–12 months and as clinically indicated *Metabolic syndrome monitoring* • Weight and BMI at 4 weeks, 8 weeks, 12 weeks, and then quarterly • Waist circumference yearly • Blood pressure at 12 weeks and then yearly • Fasting glucose (or hemoglobin A_{1C}) at 12 weeks and then yearly • Fasting lipid profile at 12 weeks and then every 5 years

Hirschfeld RMA, Bowden CL, Gitlin MJ, et al; Work Group on Bipolar Disorder: Practice Guideline for the Treatment of Patients With Bipolar Disorder, Second Edition. Washington, DC, American Psychiatric Association, 2002. Available at: http://psychiatryonline.org/pb/assets/raw/sitewide/practice_guidelines/guidelines/bipolar.pdf. Accessed May 2016; Guideline watch (November 2005): available at: http://psychiatryonline.org/pb/assets/raw/sitewide/practice_guidelines/guidelines/bipolar-watch.pdf.

Olufadi R, Byrne CD: Clinical and laboratory diagnosis of the metabolic syndrome. J Clin Pathol 61(6):697–706, 2008

Methylphenidate (Ritalin, Concerta)

Screening laboratory tests	• Electrocardiogram (ECG) and echocardiogram in patients with a family history of sudden death or ventricular arrhythmias or with physical findings suggestive of cardiovascular disease • Consider electroencephalogram (EEG) in patients with a history suggestive of seizure disorder • Pregnancy test in women who could become pregnant
Monitoring laboratory tests	• Periodic complete blood count (CBC) with differential and platelets during prolonged therapy • Prompt cardiac evaluation (ECG, echocardiogram) if syncope, exertional chest pain, or other cardiovascular symptoms develop • EEG if signs/symptoms of seizure develop • Growth rate (height) and weight measurements for children

American Society of Health-System Pharmacists: AHFS Drug Information 2016. Bethesda, MD, American Society of Health-System Pharmacists, 2016

Package Inserts. National Library of Medicine DailyMed. Available at: https://dailymed.nlm. nih.gov. Accessed May 2016.

Mirtazapine (Remeron)	
Screening laboratory tests	Although no specific laboratory testing is recommended by the manufacturer for the use of mirtazapine, the following tests should be considered: • Lipid panel to determine baseline values for later comparison • Pregnancy test in women who could become pregnant
Monitoring laboratory tests	• Periodic check of blood urea nitrogen, creatinine, estimated glomerular filtration rate, liver function tests, and lipid panel • Complete blood count if evidence of infection develops

American Society of Health-System Pharmacists: AHFS Drug Information 2016. Bethesda, MD, American Society of Health-System Pharmacists, 2016

Package Insert. National Library of Medicine DailyMed. Available at: https://dailymed.nlm. nih.gov. Accessed May 2016.

Monoamine oxidase inhibitors (MAOIs)*	
Screening laboratory tests	• Orthostatic vital signs should be checked for all patients. • Electrocardiogram for patients ≥40 years of age and for any patient with a history of cardiovascular problems • Pregnancy test in women who could become pregnant • Metabolic syndrome screening should be considered for all patients. (See Chapter 2, "Diseases and Conditions.") Other laboratory tests that may be useful include the following: • Liver function tests (LFTs) • Blood urea nitrogen, creatinine, and estimation of glomerular filtration rate • Thyroid-stimulating hormone; free thyroxine (T_4), triiodothyronine (T_3) if indicated • Fasting blood glucose (or hemoglobin A_{1C})
Monitoring laboratory tests	• Orthostatic vital signs at each visit • Periodic check of LFTs • Metabolic syndrome monitoring

*Includes isocarboxazid (Marplan), phenelzine (Nardil), and tranylcypromine (Parnate).

American Society of Health-System Pharmacists: AHFS Drug Information 2016. Bethesda, MD, American Society of Health-System Pharmacists, 2016

Package Inserts. National Library of Medicine DailyMed. Available at: https://dailymed.nlm.nih.gov. Accessed May 2016.

Naltrexone (ReVia, Vivitrol)	
Screening laboratory tests	• Blood urea nitrogen, creatinine, and estimation of glomerular filtration rate • Liver function tests (LFTs) • Hepatitis panel • Pregnancy test in women who could become pregnant
Monitoring laboratory tests	• Frequent monitoring of LFTs

American Society of Health-System Pharmacists: AHFS Drug Information 2016. Bethesda, MD, American Society of Health-System Pharmacists, 2016

Package Inserts. National Library of Medicine DailyMed. Available at: https://dailymed.nlm. nih.gov. Accessed May 2016.

Nefazodone	
Screening laboratory tests	• Liver function tests (LFTs) • Metabolic syndrome screening should be considered for all patients. (See Chapter 2, "Diseases and Conditions.")
Monitoring laboratory tests	• LFTs every 3 months • Metabolic syndrome monitoring

American Society of Health-System Pharmacists: AHFS Drug Information 2016. Bethesda, MD, American Society of Health-System Pharmacists, 2016

Package Insert. National Library of Medicine DailyMed. Available at: https://dailymed.nlm. nih.gov. Accessed May 2016.

Nonbenzodiazepine hypnotics: **eszopiclone (Lunesta), zaleplon (Sonata), zolpidem (Ambien, Edluar, Intermezzo, Zolpimist)**	
Screening laboratory tests	• Liver function tests • Pregnancy test in women who could become pregnant
Monitoring laboratory tests	• No specific laboratory monitoring is recommended by the manufacturers.

American Society of Health-System Pharmacists: AHFS Drug Information 2016. Bethesda, MD, American Society of Health-System Pharmacists, 2016

Package Inserts. National Library of Medicine DailyMed. Available at: https://dailymed.nlm. nih.gov. Accessed May 2016.

Opioids*	
Screening laboratory tests	• Blood urea nitrogen (BUN), creatinine, and estimation of glomerular filtration rate (GFR) • Liver function tests (aspartate transaminase [AST], alanine transaminase [ALT], alkaline phosphatase (ALP), bilirubin) • Amylase and lipase • Pregnancy test in women who could become pregnant
Monitoring laboratory tests	• Periodic check of BUN and creatinine, and estimation of GFR • Periodic check of AST, ALT, ALP, bilirubin • Plasma concentration of active drug may be useful in unusual or complex cases.

*Includes codeine, hydrocodone, hydromorphone, and morphine.

American Society of Health-System Pharmacists: AHFS Drug Information 2016. Bethesda, MD, American Society of Health-System Pharmacists, 2016

Package Inserts. National Library of Medicine DailyMed. Available at: https://dailymed.nlm. nih.gov. Accessed May 2016.

Oxcarbazepine (Trileptal)	
Screening laboratory tests	• Blood urea nitrogen, creatinine, and estimation of glomerular filtration rate • Serum sodium level • Pregnancy test in women who could become pregnant
Monitoring laboratory tests	• Periodic check of serum sodium level • Prompt check of serum sodium level if signs/symptoms of syndrome of inappropriate antidiuretic hormone secretion (SIADH) develop *Note:* Reductions in thyroxine (T_4) are associated with use of this drug, without concomitant changes in triiodothyronine (T_3) or thyroid-stimulating hormone; thyroid monitoring is not required.

American Society of Health-System Pharmacists: AHFS Drug Information 2016. Bethesda, MD, American Society of Health-System Pharmacists, 2016

Package Insert. National Library of Medicine DailyMed. Available at: https://dailymed.nlm. nih.gov. Accessed May 2016.

Ramelteon (Rozerem)	
Screening laboratory tests	• Liver function tests • Polysomnography may be indicated for patients with suspected sleep apnea. • Pregnancy test in women who could become pregnant
Monitoring laboratory tests	• No standard monitoring is recommended by the manufacturer. • For patients presenting with unexplained amenorrhea, galactorrhea, decreased libido, or problems with fertility, assessment of prolactin levels and testosterone levels should be considered, as appropriate.

American Society of Health-System Pharmacists: AHFS Drug Information 2016. Bethesda, MD, American Society of Health-System Pharmacists, 2016

Package Insert. National Library of Medicine DailyMed. Available at: https://dailymed.nlm. nih.gov. Accessed May 2016.

Rivastigmine (Exelon)	
Screening laboratory tests	• Blood urea nitrogen (BUN) and creatinine and estimation of glomerular filtration rate (GFR) • Liver function tests (LFTs) • Consider electrocardiogram (ECG) to exclude supraventricular conduction abnormalities • Pregnancy test in women who could become pregnant
Monitoring laboratory tests	• Periodic check of BUN and creatinine and estimation of GFR • Periodic check of LFTs • ECG in the event of clinical evidence of atrial fibrillation, bradycardia, or other cardiac abnormality • Monitor weight changes to determine whether dosage adjustment is indicated.

American Society of Health-System Pharmacists: AHFS Drug Information 2016. Bethesda, MD, American Society of Health-System Pharmacists, 2016

Package Insert. U.S. National Library of Medicine DailyMed. Available at: https://dailymed.nlm.nih.gov. Accessed May 2016.

Selective serotonin reuptake inhibitors (SSRIs)*	
Screening laboratory tests	• Serum sodium • Metabolic syndrome screening should be considered for all patients. (See Chapter 2, "Diseases and Conditions.") • Pregnancy test in women who could become pregnant

Monitoring laboratory tests	• Periodic checks of the following:
	
	   • Serum sodium
	
	   • Liver function
	
	   • Pulse, with electrocardiogram performed if abnormal
	
	• Metabolic syndrome monitoring

*Includes citalopram, escitalopram, fluoxetine, fluvoxamine, paroxetine, sertraline, and vortioxetine.

American Society of Health-System Pharmacists: AHFS Drug Information 2016. Bethesda, MD, American Society of Health-System Pharmacists, 2016

Package Inserts. National Library of Medicine DailyMed. Available at: https://dailymed.nlm. nih.gov. Accessed May 2016.

Topiramate (Topamax)	
Screening laboratory tests	• Blood urea nitrogen (BUN) and creatinine and estimation of glomerular filtration rate (GFR) • Electrolyte panel or metabolic panel (basic or comprehensive) to check bicarbonate level • Pregnancy test in women who could become pregnant
Monitoring laboratory tests	• BUN and creatinine and estimation of GFR periodically during treatment • Periodic check of bicarbonate level • Ammonia level in patients who develop confusion or delirium, especially those coadministered valproate • Clinical evidence of acute visual disturbance or myopia

American Society of Health-System Pharmacists: AHFS Drug Information 2016. Bethesda, MD, American Society of Health-System Pharmacists, 2016

Package Insert. National Library of Medicine DailyMed. Available at: https://dailymed.nlm. nih.gov. Accessed May 2016.

Tramadol (Ultram)	
Screening laboratory tests	• Blood urea nitrogen and creatinine and estimation of glomerular filtration rate to determine the need for dosage adjustment • Liver function tests to determine the need for dosage adjustment • Electroencephalogram (EEG) should be considered in patients with a history suggestive of seizure disorder. • Pregnancy test in women who could become pregnant
Monitoring laboratory tests	• No routine monitoring is recommended by the manufacturer. • EEG should be considered in any patient who develops signs/ symptoms suggestive of seizure.

American Society of Health-System Pharmacists: AHFS Drug Information 2016. Bethesda, MD, American Society of Health-System Pharmacists, 2016

Package Insert. National Library of Medicine DailyMed. Available at: https://dailymed.nlm. nih.gov. Accessed May 2016.

Trazodone (Desyrel, Oleptro)	
Screening laboratory tests	• White blood cell count (WBC) and absolute neutrophil count (ANC) • Serum sodium, especially in geriatric patients • Blood urea nitrogen and creatinine and estimation of glomerular filtration rate • Liver function tests • Electrocardiogram (ECG) in patients with cardiovascular disease • Orthostatic vital signs • Pregnancy test in women who could become pregnant
Monitoring laboratory tests	• WBC and ANC check when fever and sore throat or other signs of infection develop during therapy • Orthostatic vital signs • Re-check of baseline labs and ECG as clinically indicated

American Society of Health-System Pharmacists: AHFS Drug Information 2016. Bethesda, MD, American Society of Health-System Pharmacists, 2016

Package Inserts. National Library of Medicine DailyMed. Available at: https://dailymed.nlm. nih.gov. Accessed May 2016.

Tricyclic antidepressants (TCAs)*	
Screening laboratory tests	When TCAs are prescribed to treat depression, laboratory tests are performed to exclude medical conditions that could underlie the presentation (e.g., anemia, hypothyroidism, vitamin B_{12} deficiency), complicate treatment (e.g., heart block or renal insufficiency), or contribute to poor treatment response (e.g., folate deficiency). In addition, regardless of the indication, "safety labs" are required, particularly when TCAs are used in elderly or other medically vulnerable patients. Monitoring for the metabolic syndrome is indicated if long-term treatment is needed. Screening laboratory tests typically include the following: • Complete blood count • Electrolytes (potassium, calcium, sodium, magnesium) • Blood urea nitrogen and creatinine • Liver function tests • Vitamin B_{12} level • Red blood cell folate level • Thyroid-stimulating hormone • Electrocardiogram (ECG) for patients ≥40 years and for any patient with a history of cardiac problems • Pregnancy test in women who could become pregnant *Metabolic syndrome screening* • Fasting glucose • Fasting lipid profile • Weight, height, body mass index (BMI) calculation • Waist circumference • Blood pressure
Monitoring laboratory tests	• When TCA drug levels are checked, blood should be drawn when steady state has been reached, 12 hours after the last dose (trough level). • ECG at steady state • ECG yearly thereafter; more often for any patient with a history of cardiac problems • ECG for suspected TCA toxicity

Tricyclic antidepressants (TCAs)* *(continued)*	
Monitoring laboratory tests *(continued)*	*Metabolic syndrome monitoring* • Weight and BMI at 4 weeks, 8 weeks, 12 weeks, and then quarterly • Waist circumference yearly • Blood pressure at 12 weeks and then yearly • Fasting glucose at 12 weeks and then yearly • Fasting lipid profile at 12 weeks and then every 5 years

*Includes amitriptyline, clomipramine, desipramine, doxepin, imipramine, and nortriptyline.

American Society of Health-System Pharmacists: AHFS Drug Information 2016. Bethesda, MD, American Society of Health-System Pharmacists, 2016

Package Inserts. National Library of Medicine DailyMed. Available at: https://dailymed.nlm. nih.gov. Accessed May 2016.

Valproate	
Screening laboratory tests	• Complete blood count (CBC) with platelets • Liver function tests (LFTs) • Thyroid-stimulating hormone (TSH) • Pregnancy test in women who could become pregnant *Metabolic syndrome screening* • Fasting glucose • Fasting lipid profile • Weight, height, body mass index (BMI) calculation • Waist circumference • Blood pressure
Monitoring laboratory tests	• CBC with platelets and LFTs every week during initial drug titration • CBC with platelets, LFTs, serum ammonia, TSH, amylase, and lipase every 6 months thereafter • Valproate level as needed to check noncompliance or toxicity *Metabolic syndrome monitoring* • Weight and BMI at 4 weeks, 8 weeks, 12 weeks, and then quarterly • Waist circumference yearly • Blood pressure at 12 weeks and then yearly • Fasting glucose at 12 weeks and then yearly • Fasting lipid profile at 12 weeks and then every 5 years

American Society of Health-System Pharmacists: AHFS Drug Information 2016. Bethesda, MD, American Society of Health-System Pharmacists, 2016

Package Insert. National Library of Medicine DailyMed. Available at: https://dailymed.nlm. nih.gov. Accessed June 2016.

Venlafaxine (Effexor); desvenlafaxine (Pristiq)	
Screening laboratory tests	When these medications are prescribed to treat depression or anxiety, laboratory tests are performed to exclude medical conditions that could underlie the presentation (e.g., anemia, thyroid dysfunction, vitamin B_{12} deficiency), complicate treatment (e.g., renal insufficiency), or contribute to poor treatment response (e.g., folate deficiency).
	Although no specific laboratory testing is recommended by the manufacturer for the use of venlafaxine or desvenlafaxine, the following tests should be considered:
	• Electrocardiogram for patients ≥40 years and for any patient with a history of cardiac problems
	• Lipid panel
	• Pregnancy test in women who could become pregnant
Monitoring laboratory tests	• Periodic check of electrolytes, blood urea nitrogen, creatinine, liver function tests, and lipid panel may show changes pertinent to the long-term use of these medications.

American Society of Health-System Pharmacists: AHFS Drug Information 2016. Bethesda, MD, American Society of Health-System Pharmacists, 2016

Package Inserts. National Library of Medicine DailyMed. Available at: https://dailymed.nlm. nih.gov. Accessed June 2016.

Appendix

Therapeutic and toxic drug levels at a glance

Drug	Therapeutic level (trough)	Toxic level (random)
Amitriptyline (+nortriptyline)	80–200 ng/mL	≥300 ng/mL
Amoxapine (+ 8-hydroamoxapine)	200–400 ng/mL	*
Aripiprazole	109–585 ng/mL[#]	*
Carbamazepine, total	4–12 µg/mL	≥15 µg/mL
Carbamazepine, free	1–3 µg/mL	≥4 µg/mL
Clozapine	>350 ng/mL	>1,200 ng/mL
Clozapine (+norclozapine)	>450 ng/mL	
Desipramine	100–300 ng/mL	≥300 ng/mL
Doxepin (+nordoxepin)	50–150 ng/mL	≥300 ng/mL
Haloperidol	5–16 ng/mL	*
Reduced haloperidol	10–80 ng/mL	
Imipramine (+desipramine)	175–300 ng/mL	>300 ng/mL
Lamotrigine	2.5–15 µg/mL	>20 µg/mL
Levetiracetam	12–46 µg/mL	*
Lithium	0.5–1.2 mmol/L	≥1.6 mmol/L
Nortriptyline	70–170 ng/mL	≥300 ng/mL
Olanzapine	10–80 ng/mL[#]	*
Perphenazine	5–30 ng/mL (0.5–2.5 ng/mL for low-dose therapy)	*
Phenytoin, total	10–20 µg/mL	≥30 µg/mL
Phenytoin, free	1–2 µg/mL	≥2.5 µg/mL
Percent free phenytoin	8%–14% (calculated)	
Quetiapine	100–1,000 ng/mL[#]	*
Risperidone (+ 9-OH-risperidone)	10–120 ng/mL[#]	*
Thiothixene	10–30 ng/mL	*
Trazodone	800–1,600 ng/mL	*
Valproate, total	50 (trough)–125 (peak) µg/mL	≥151 µg/mL
Valproate, free	5–25 µg/mL	>30 µg/mL
Percent free valproate	5%–18% (calculated)	
Ziprasidone	Up to 220 ng/mL[#]	*

*Range not well established. #Denotes expected steady state levels in patients receiving recommended dosages (not therapeutic ranges).

Source.   Mayo Clinic, Mayo Medical Laboratories Test Catalog. Available at: http://www.mayo-medicallaboratories.com. Accessed July 2016.

Ten rules for a normal electrocardiogram

1. The PR interval should be 120–200 milliseconds (3–5 small squares).

2. The QRS complex should not be wider than 110 milliseconds (<3 small squares).

3. The QRS complex should be mostly upright in leads I and II.

4. The QRS and T waves should have the same general polarity (up or down) in limb leads.

5. All waves in aVR are downgoing (negative).

6. The R wave should grow across precordial leads (V_1 to V_6), at least to V_4.

7. The ST segment should start at baseline (be isoelectric) in all leads except V_1 and V_2, where it may start above the baseline.

8. P waves should be upright in leads I, II, and V_2 to V_6.

9. Q waves should be absent, except for small Q waves of <0.04 seconds in I, II, and V_2 to V_6.

10. The T wave must be upright in I, II, and V_2 to V_6.

Source. Douglas Chamberlain, M.D., F.R.C.P., Brighton and Sussex Medical School, University of Brighton, United Kingdom. Used with permission.

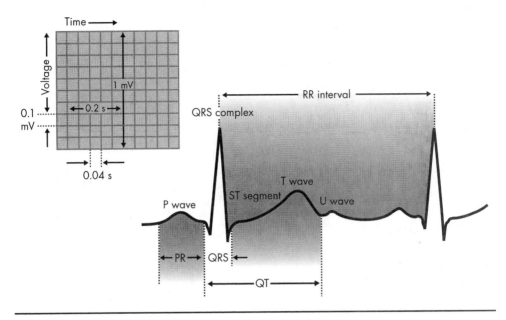

Figure 1. The electrocardiogram: waves and intervals.

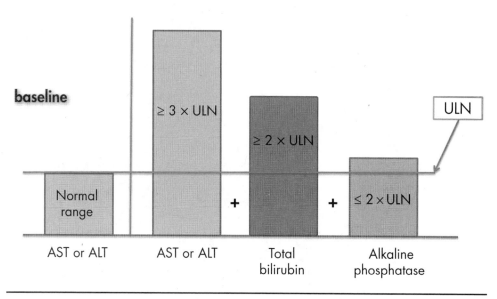

Figure 2. Hy's law.

Hy's law (or Hy's criteria) helps to identify hepatotoxic drugs and drug reactions. Baseline values of aspartate transaminase (AST) or alanine transaminase (ALT) are in the normal range. After the drug is started (*vertical line*): AST or ALT≥3× ULN (liver injury); total bilirubin (BR)≥2× ULN (enough to impair capacity to excrete BR); no evidence of an obstructive pattern (no elevation in alkaline phosphatase) and no other reason for liver injury. ULN=upper limit of normal.

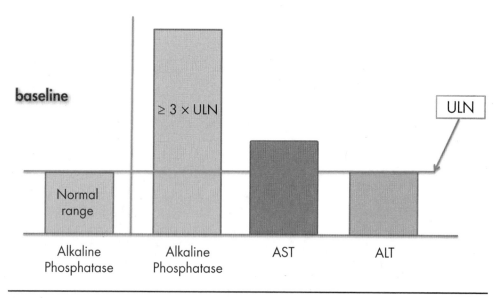

Figure 3. Cholestatic injury.

A cholestatic drug reaction is suggested by an increase in alkaline phosphatase, usually greater than three times the upper limit of normal. Aspartate transaminase (AST) and alanine transaminase (ALT) levels are normal or only minimally elevated.

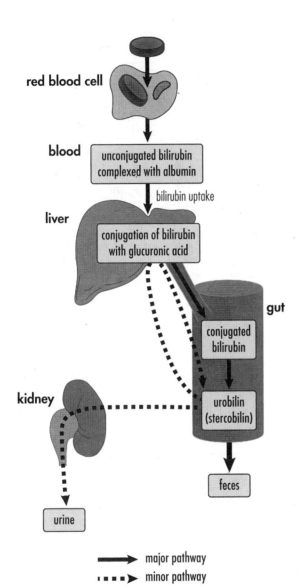

Bilirubin is derived mainly from red blood cell (hemoglobin) breakdown. This is unconjugated bilirubin. It travels with albumin to the liver.

In the liver, bilirubin is conjugated with glucuronic acid, making it water-soluble. It can then be excreted in feces and urine.

Prehepatic disease such as hemolytic anemia causes increased unconjugated bilirubin.

Posthepatic disease such as bile duct obstruction causes increased conjugated bilirubin.

Liver disease such as hepatitis causes increased conjugated and unconjugated bilirubin.

Figure 4. Bilirubin cycle.
Red blood cell breakdown gives rise to bilirubin in the circulation, which binds to albumin and travels to the liver. There, bilirubin is conjugated with glucuronic acid and secreted into bile and then to the gastrointestinal tract. In the gut, the glucuronic acid is removed and the bilirubin is converted to urobilinogen and then to the brown-colored stercobilin.

(A)

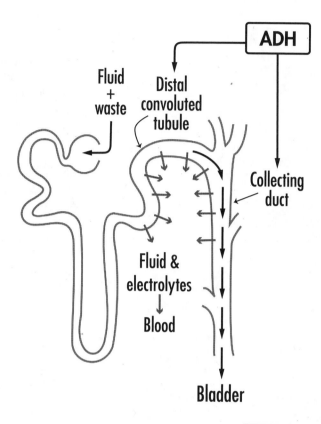

(B)

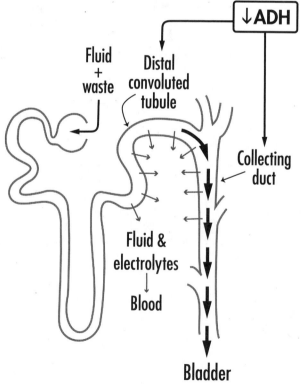

(C)

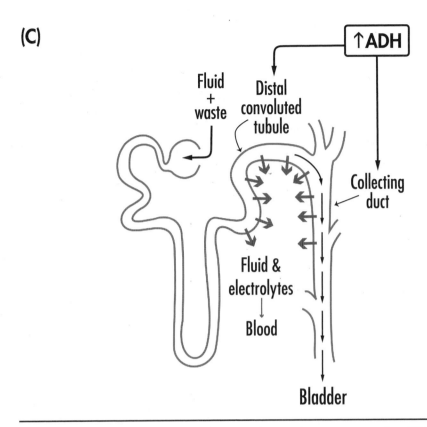

Figure 5. Syndrome of inappropriate antidiuretic hormone secretion (SIADH).
(A) Antidiuretic hormone (ADH) acts on the nephron, which controls water excretion.
(B) When serum ADH level is decreased, the nephron excretes water.
(C) When serum ADH level is increased, the nephron retains water. Serum becomes dilute, while urine becomes concentrated. At the same time, serum sodium decreases and urine sodium increases. Under normal conditions, a drop in serum osmolality signals osmoreceptors in the hypothalamus to reduce ADH secretion. In certain conditions and with certain drugs, however, ADH continues to be secreted when serum osmolality is low. This is the syndrome of inappropriate ADH secretion, or SIADH, in which serum osmolality is low, urine osmolality is high, serum sodium is low, and urine sodium is high.

References

Adrogué HJ, Madias NE: Hyponatremia. N Engl J Med 342(21):1581–1589, 2000 10824078

Agarwal N, Port JD, Bazzocchi M, Renshaw PF: Update on the use of MR for assessment and diagnosis of psychiatric diseases. Radiology 255(1):23–41, 2010 20308442

Ahmed MH: Biochemical markers: the road map for the diagnosis of nonalcoholic fatty liver disease. Am J Clin Pathol 127(1):20–22, 2007 17145635

American College of Endocrinology and American Diabetes Association: Consensus statement on inpatient diabetes and glycemic control. Diabetes Care 29:1955–1962, 2006

American Psychiatric Association: Diagnostic and Statistical Manual of Mental Disorders, 4th Edition, Text Revision. Washington, DC, American Psychiatric Association, 2000a

American Psychiatric Association: Practice Guidelines for the Treatment of Psychiatric Disorders. Washington, DC, American Psychiatric Association, 2000b

American Psychiatric Association: Practice guideline for the treatment of patients with schizophrenia, second edition. Am J Psychiatry 161(2, Suppl):1–56, 2004

American Psychiatric Association: Diagnostic and Statistical Manual of Mental Disorders, 5th Edition. Arlington, VA, American Psychiatric Association, 2013

American Society of Health-System Pharmacists: AHFS Drug Information. Bethesda, MD, American Society of Health-System Pharmacists, 2016

ARUP Laboratories: Laboratory Test Directory. Available at: http://www.aruplab.com. Accessed May 2010.

Barceloux DG, Krenzelok EP, Olson K, Watson W; Ad Hoc Committee: American Academy of Clinical Toxicology practice guidelines on the treatment of ethylene glycol poisoning. J Toxicol Clin Toxicol 37(5):537–560, 1999 10497633

Bart G, Piccolo P, Zhang L, et al: Markers for hepatitis A, B and C in methadone maintained patients: an unexpectedly high co-infection with silent hepatitis B. Addiction 103(4):681–686, 2008 18339114

Baskin HJ, Cobin RH, Duick DS, et al; American Association of Clinical Endocrinologists: American Association of Clinical Endocrinologists medical guidelines for clinical practice for the evaluation and treatment of hyperthyroidism and hypothyroidism. Endocr Pract 8(6):457–469, 2002 15260011

Beck FK, Rosenthal TC: Prealbumin: a marker for nutritional evaluation. Am Fam Physician 65(8):1575–1578, 2002 11989633

Benes H, Walters AS, Allen RP, et al: Definition of restless legs syndrome, how to diagnose it, and how to differentiate it from RLS mimics. Mov Disord 22 (Suppl 18):S401–S408, 2007

Biondi B, Palmieri EA, Klain M, et al: Subclinical hyperthyroidism: clinical features and treatment options. Eur J Endocrinol 152(1):1–9, 2005 15762182

Boldt J: Use of albumin: an update. Br J Anaesth 104(3):276–284, 2010 20100698

Brent J: Current management of ethylene glycol poisoning. Drugs 61(7):979–988, 2001 11434452

Brewster UC, Perazella MA: A review of chronic lead intoxication: an unrecognized cause of chronic kidney disease. Am J Med Sci 327(6):341–347, 2004

Brodie D, Schluger NW: The diagnosis of tuberculosis. Clin Chest Med 26:247–271, vi, 2005

Brown JS: Environmental and Chemical Toxins and Psychiatric Illness. Washington, DC, American Psychiatric Publishing, 2002

Brunzell JD: Clinical practice. Hypertriglyceridemia. N Engl J Med 357(10):1009–1017, 2007 17804845

Brust JC: A 74-year-old man with memory loss and neuropathy who enjoys alcoholic beverages. JAMA 299(9):1046–1054, 2008 18252872

Buxbaum JD: Multiple rare variants in the etiology of autism spectrum disorders. Dialogues Clin Neurosci 11:35–43, 2009

Cain KP, McCarthy KD, Heilig CM, et al: An algorithm for tuberculosis screening and diagnosis in people with HIV. N Engl J Med 362(8):707–716, 2010 20181972

Catafau AM: Brain SPECT in clinical practice. Part I: perfusion. J Nucl Med 42(2):259–271, 2001 11216525

Chen DK, So YT, Fisher RS; Therapeutics and Technology Assessment Subcommittee of the American Academy of Neurology: Use of serum prolactin in diagnosing epileptic seizures: report of the Therapeutics and Technology Assessment Subcommittee of the American Academy of Neurology. Neurology 65(5):668–675, 2005 16157897

Chrostek L, Cylwik B, Szmitkowski M, Korcz W: The diagnostic accuracy of carbohydrate-deficient transferrin, sialic acid and commonly used markers of alcohol abuse during abstinence. Clin Chim Acta 364(1-2):167–171, 2006 16087169

Clyne B, Jerrard DA: Syphilis testing. J Emerg Med 18(3):361–367, 2000 10729677

Cohn RM, Roth KS: Hyperammonemia, bane of the brain. Clin Pediatr (Phila) 43(8):683–689, 2004 15494874

Col NF, Surks MI, Daniels GH: Subclinical thyroid disease: clinical applications. JAMA 291(2):239–243, 2004 14722151

Corathers SD: Focus on diagnosis: the alkaline phosphatase level: nuances of a familiar test. Pediatr Rev 27(10):382–384, 2006 17012488

Costabel U, Ohshimo S, Guzman J: Diagnosis of sarcoidosis. Curr Opin Pulm Med 14(5):455–461, 2008

de Leon J, Armstrong SC, Cozza KL: Clinical guidelines for psychiatrists for the use of pharmacogenetic testing for CYP450 2D6 and CYP450 2C19. Psychosomatics 47(1):75–85, 2006 16384813

Descombes E, Dessibourg CA, Fellay G: Acute encephalopathy due to thiamine deficiency (Wernicke's encephalopathy) in a chronic hemodialyzed patient: a case report. Clin Nephrol 35(4):171–175, 1991 1855320

Dørup I: Magnesium and potassium deficiency. Its diagnosis, occurrence and treatment in diuretic therapy and its consequences for growth, protein synthesis and growth factors. Acta Physiol Scand Suppl 618:1–55, 1994 8036903

Dundas B, Harris M, Narasimhan M: Psychogenic polydipsia review: etiology, differential, and treatment. Curr Psychiatry Rep 9(3):236–241, 2007 17521521

Dyckner T, Wester PO: Magnesium deficiency: guidelines for diagnosis and substitution therapy. Acta Med Scand Suppl 661:37–41, 1982 6959478

Ellison DH, Berl T: Clinical practice. The syndrome of inappropriate antidiuresis. N Engl J Med 356(20):2064–2072, 2007 17507705

Evaluation of Genomic Applications in Practice and Prevention (EGAPP) Working Group: Recommendations from the EGAPP Working Group: testing for cytochrome P450 polymorphisms in adults with nonpsychotic depression treated with selective serotonin reuptake inhibitors. Genet Med 9(12):819–825, 2007 18091431

Factora R, Luciano M: When to consider normal pressure hydrocephalus in the patient with gait disturbance. Geriatrics 63(2):32–37, 2008 18312021

Fauci AS, Braunwald E, Kasper DL, et al (eds): Harrison's Principles of Internal Medicine, 17th Edition. New York, McGraw-Hill, 2008

Fischbach F, Dunning MB: A Manual of Laboratory and Diagnostic Tests, 8th Edition. Philadelphia, PA, Wolters Kluwer Health/Lippincott Williams & Wilkins, 2009

Flemons WW: Clinical practice. Obstructive sleep apnea. N Engl J Med 347(7):498–504, 2002 12181405

Franken WP, Timmermans JF, Prins C, et al: Comparison of Mantoux and QuantiFERON TB Gold tests for diagnosis of latent tuberculosis infection in Army personnel. Clin Vaccine Immunol 14(4):477–480, 2007 17301213

Frankenburg FR: Alcohol use, thiamine deficiency, and cognitive impairment. JAMA 299:2854, author reply 2854–2855, 2008

Freeman ME, Kanyicska B, Lerant A, Nagy G: Prolactin: structure, function, and regulation of secretion. Physiol Rev 80(4):1523–1631, 2000 11015620

Fuhrman MP, Charney P, Mueller CM: Hepatic proteins and nutrition assessment. J Am Diet Assoc 104(8):1258–1264, 2004 15281044

Galanter M, Kleber HD, Brady KT (eds): The American Psychiatric Publishing Textbook of Substance Abuse Treatment, 5th Edition. Arlington, VA, American Psychiatric Publishing, 2015

Gans DA: Biochemical measures of thiamine deficiency. Am J Clin Nutr 65(4):1090–1092, 1997 9094901

Garton HJ, Piatt JH Jr: Hydrocephalus. Pediatr Clin North Am 51(2):305–325, 2004 15062673

Germon K: Fluid and electrolyte problems associated with diabetes insipidus and syndrome of inappropriate antidiuretic hormone. Nurs Clin North Am 22(4):785–796, 1987 3317286

Ghio L, Fornaro G, Rossi P: Risperidone-induced hyperamylasemia, hyperlipasemia, and neuro-leptic malignant syndrome: a case report. J Clin Psychopharmacol 29(4):391–392, 2009 19593182

Giannini EG, Testa R, Savarino V: Liver enzyme alteration: a guide for clinicians. CMAJ 172(3):367–379, 2005 15684121

Gopal DV, Rosen HR: Abnormal findings on liver function tests: interpreting results to narrow the diagnosis and establish a prognosis. Postgrad Med 107:100–102, 105–109, 113–114, 2000

Hales RE, Yudofsky SC, Roberts LW (eds): The American Psychiatric Publishing Textbook of Psychiatry, 6th Edition. Arlington, VA, American Psychiatric Publishing, 2014

Hanly JG, Urowitz MB, Siannis F, et al; Systemic Lupus International Collaborating Clinics: Autoantibodies and neuropsychiatric events at the time of systemic lupus erythematosus diagnosis: results from an international inception cohort study. Arthritis Rheum 58(3):843–853, 2008 18311802

Herholz K, Carter SF, Jones M: Positron emission tomography imaging in dementia. Br J Radiol 80(Spec No 2):S160–S167, 2007 18445746

Hirschfeld RMA, Bowden CL, Gitlin MJ, et al; Work Group on Bipolar Disorder: Practice Guideline for the Treatment of Patients With Bipolar Disorder, 2nd Edition. Washington, DC, American Psychiatric Association, 2002. Available at: http://psychiatryonline.org/pb/assets/raw/sitewide/practice_guidelines/guidelines/bipolar.pdf. Accessed May 2016. Guideline watch (November 2005); available at: http://psychiatryonline.org/pb/assets/raw/sitewide/practice_guidelines/guidelines/bipolar-watch.pdf.

Holt RE: The role of computed tomography of the brain in psychiatry. Psychiatr Med 1(3):275–285, 1983 6599851

Hvas AM, Nexo E: Diagnosis and treatment of vitamin B$_{12}$ deficiency—an update. Haematologica 91(11):1506–1512, 2006 17043022

Iglesias P, Dévora O, García J, et al: Severe hyperthyroidism: aetiology, clinical features and treatment outcome. Clin Endocrinol (Oxf) 72(4):551–557, 2010 19681915

Irani DN: Cerebrospinal Fluid in Clinical Practice. Philadelphia, PA, Saunders Elsevier, 2009

Jacobson SA: Delirium in the elderly. Psychiatr Clin North Am 20(1):91–110, 1997 9139298

Jacobson SA, Pies RW, Katz IR: Clinical Manual of Geriatric Psychopharmacology. Washington, DC, American Psychiatric Publishing, 2007

Jacobson S, Jerrier H: EEG in delirium. Semin Clin Neuropsychiatry 5(2):86–92, 2000 10837097

Johnston DE: Special considerations in interpreting liver function tests. Am Fam Physician 59(8):2223–2230, 1999 10221307

Judson MA: The diagnosis of sarcoidosis. Clin Chest Med 29(3):415–427, viii, 2008

Kasper DL, Fauci AS, Hauser SL, et al (eds): Harrison's Principles of Internal Medicine, 19th Edition. New York, McGraw-Hill, 2015

Katz KD, Brooks DE: Toxicity, Organophosphate. eMedicine. Available at: http://emedicine.medscape.com/article/167726. Accessed October 2010.

Katz U, Zandman-Goddard G: Drug-induced lupus: an update. Autoimmun Rev 10(1):46–50, 2010 20656071

Kim JM, Stewart R, Kim SW, et al: Predictive value of folate, vitamin B$_{12}$ and homocysteine levels in late-life depression. Br J Psychiatry 192(4):268–274, 2008 18378986

Kraut JA, Kurtz I: Toxic alcohol ingestions: clinical features, diagnosis, and management. Clin J Am Soc Nephrol 3(1):208–225, 2008 18045860

Kundra A, Jain A, Banga A, et al: Evaluation of plasma ammonia levels in patients with acute liver failure and chronic liver disease and its correlation with the severity of hepatic encephalopathy and clinical features of raised intracranial tension. Clin Biochem 38(8):696–699, 2005 15963970

Leiken SJ, Caplan H: Psychogenic polydipsia. Am J Psychiatry 123(12):1573–1576, 1967 6025192

Lerner V, Kanevsky M, Dwolatzky T, et al: Vitamin B$_{12}$ and folate serum levels in newly admitted psychiatric patients. Clin Nutr 25(1):60–67, 2006 16216392

Levey AS, Bosch JP, Lewis JB, et al; Modification of Diet in Renal Disease Study Group: A more accurate method to estimate glomerular filtration rate from serum creatinine: a new prediction equation. Ann Intern Med 130(6):461–470, 1999 10075613

Lidofsky SD: Nonalcoholic fatty liver disease: diagnosis and relation to metabolic syndrome and approach to treatment. Curr Diab Rep 8(1):25–30, 2008 18366995

Lien YH, Shapiro JI: Hyponatremia: clinical diagnosis and management. Am J Med 120(8):653–658, 2007 17679119

Lin YH, Wang Y, Loua A, et al: Evaluation of a new hepatitis B virus surface antigen rapid test with improved sensitivity. J Clin Microbiol 46(10):3319–3324, 2008 18701669

Lintas C, Persico AM: Autistic phenotypes and genetic testing: state-of-the-art for the clinical geneticist. J Med Genet 46:1–8, 2009

Mayo Clinic: Mayo Medical Laboratories Test Catalog. Available at: http://www.mayomedicallaboratories.com/test-catalog/. Accessed May–August 2016.

McConnell LM, Sanders GD, Owens DK: Evaluation of genetic tests: APOE genotyping for the diagnosis of Alzheimer disease. Genet Test 3(1):47–53, 1999 10464577

Meltzer HY, Cola PA, Parsa M: Marked elevations of serum creatine kinase activity associated with antipsychotic drug treatment. Neuropsychopharmacology 15(4):395–405, 1996 8887994

Misdraji J, Nguyen PL: Urinalysis. When—and when not—to order. Postgrad Med 100(1):173–176, 181–182, 185–188 passim, 1996 8668615

Misra M, Papakostas GI, Klibanski A: Effects of psychiatric disorders and psychotropic medications on prolactin and bone metabolism. J Clin Psychiatry 65:1607–1618, quiz 1590, 1760–1761, 2004

Moeller KE, Lee KC, Kissack JC: Urine drug screening: practical guide for clinicians. Mayo Clin Proc 83(1):66–76, 2008 18174009

Mohri I, Kato-Nishimura K, Tachibana N, et al: Restless legs syndrome (RLS): an unrecognized cause for bedtime problems and insomnia in children. Sleep Med 9(6):701–702, 2008

Moore DP, Jefferson JW: Handbook of Medical Psychiatry, 2nd Edition. Philadelphia, PA, Elsevier/Mosby, 2004

Morris J, Twaddle S: Anorexia nervosa. BMJ 334(7599):894–898, 2007 17463461

Mosconi L, Tsui WH, Herholz K, et al: Multicenter standardized 18F-FDG PET diagnosis of mild cognitive impairment, Alzheimer's disease, and other dementias. J Nucl Med 49(3):390–398, 2008 18287270

Moyer VA; U.S. Preventive Services Task Force: Screening for HIV: U.S. Preventive Services Task Force Recommendation Statement. Ann Intern Med 159(1):51–60, 2013 23698354

Mulholland PJ: Susceptibility of the cerebellum to thiamine deficiency. Cerebellum 5(1):55–63, 2006 16527765

Myers RP: Noninvasive diagnosis of nonalcoholic fatty liver disease. Ann Hepatol 8(Suppl 1):S25–S33, 2009 19381121

National Cholesterol Education Program (NCEP) Expert Panel on Detection, Evaluation, and Treatment of High Blood Cholesterol in Adults (Adult Treatment Panel III): Third Report of the National Cholesterol Education Program (NCEP) Expert Panel on Detection, Evaluation, and Treatment of High Blood Cholesterol in Adults (Adult Treatment Panel III) final report. Circulation 106(25):3143–3421, 2002 12485966

National Guideline Clearinghouse: ACR Appropriateness Criteria. Available at: http://www.ngc.gov. Accessed May 2010.

National Institutes of Health: Consensus Statement on Management of Hepatitis C: 2002. NIH Consens State Sci Statements 19:1–46, 2002

O'Keeffe ST: Thiamine deficiency in elderly people. Age Ageing 29(2):99–101, 2000 10791442

Olufadi R, Byrne CD: Clinical and laboratory diagnosis of the metabolic syndrome. J Clin Pathol 61(6):697–706, 2008 18505888

Otsuka: Brexiprazole (package insert). Available at: https://www.otsuka-us.com/media/static/Rexulti-PI.pdf.Accessed June 10, 2016.

Package Inserts. National Library of Medicine DailyMed. Available at: http://dailymed.nlm.nih.gov/dailymed. Accessed May–June, September 2016.

Park SY, Jeon K, Um SW, et al: Clinical utility of the QuantiFERON-TB Gold In-Tube test for the diagnosis of active pulmonary tuberculosis. Scand J Infect Dis 41(11-12):818–822, 2009 19922063

Parrish S, Turner JF: Diagnosis of sarcoidosis. Dis Mon 55(11):693–703, 2009

Patel P, Macerollo A: Diabetes mellitus: diagnosis and screening. Am Fam Physician 81(7):863–870, 2010 20353144

Petersen RC, Waring SC, Smith GE, et al: Predictive value of APOE genotyping in incipient Alzheimer's disease. Ann N Y Acad Sci 802:58–69, 1996 8993485

Phypers M, Harris T, Power C: CNS tuberculosis: a longitudinal analysis of epidemiological and clinical features. Int J Tuberc Lung Dis 10(1):99–103, 2006 16466045

Piana F, Ruffo Codecasa L, Baldan R, et al: Use of T-SPOT.TB in latent tuberculosis infection diagnosis in general and immunosuppressed populations. New Microbiol 30(3):286–290, 2007 17802911

Price RW, Epstein LG, Becker JT, et al: Biomarkers of HIV-1 CNS infection and injury. Neurology 69(18):1781–1788, 2007 17967994

Rack M, Davis J, Roffwarg HP, et al: The multiple sleep latency test in the diagnosis of narcolepsy. Am J Psychiatry 162:2198–2199, author reply 2199, 2005

Rao SN, Chandak GR: Cardiac beriberi: often a missed diagnosis. J Trop Pediatr 56(4):284–285, 2010 19934228

Record CO: Neurochemistry of hepatic encephalopathy. Gut 32(11):1261–1263, 1991 1752451

Reisfield GM, Bertholf RL: "Practical guide" to urine drug screening clarified. Mayo Clin Proc 83:848–849, author reply 849, 2008

Reust CE, Hall L: Clinical inquiries. What is the differential diagnosis of an elevated alkaline phosphatase (AP) level in an otherwise asymptomatic patient? J Fam Pract 50(6):496–497, 2001 11401735

Reynolds RM, Padfield PL, Seckl JR: Disorders of sodium balance. BMJ 332(7543):702–705, 2006 16565125

Rinck D, Frieling H, Freitag A, et al: Combinations of carbohydrate-deficient transferrin, mean corpuscular erythrocyte volume, gamma-glutamyltransferase, homocysteine and folate increase the significance of biological markers in alcohol dependent patients. Drug Alcohol Depend 89(1):60–65, 2007 17234365

Roberts CG, Ladenson PW: Hypothyroidism. Lancet 363(9411):793–803, 2004 15016491

Robinson AG: Disorders of antidiuretic hormone secretion. Clin Endocrinol Metab 14(1):55–88, 1985 3893810

Rosebush PI, Anglin RE, Richards C, Mazurek MF: Neuroleptic malignant syndrome and the acute phase response. J Clin Psychopharmacol 28(4):459–461, 2008 18626278

Rosse RB, Giese AA, Deutsch SI, et al: A Concise Guide to Laboratory and Diagnostic Testing in Psychiatry. Washington, DC, American Psychiatric Publishing, 1989

Royer M, Castelo-Branco C, Blümel JE, et al; Collaborative Group for Research of the Climacteric in Latin America: The US National Cholesterol Education Programme Adult Treatment Panel III (NCEP ATP III): prevalence of the metabolic syndrome in postmenopausal Latin American women. Climacteric 10(2):164–170, 2007 17453865

Rushing JM, Jones LE, Carney CP: Bulimia nervosa: a primary care review. Prim Care Companion J Clin Psychiatry 5(5):217–224, 2003 15213788

Saudek CD, Derr RL, Kalyani RR: Assessing glycemia in diabetes using self-monitoring blood glucose and hemoglobin A1c. JAMA 295(14):1688–1697, 2006 16609091

Saxena K: Clinical features and management of poisoning due to potassium chloride. Med Toxicol 4(6):429–443, 1989 2689836

Sechi G, Serra A: Wernicke's encephalopathy: new clinical settings and recent advances in diagnosis and management. Lancet Neurol 6(5):442–455, 2007 17434099

Shulman DI, Muhar I, Jorgensen EV, et al: Autoimmune hyperthyroidism in prepubertal children and adolescents: comparison of clinical and biochemical features at diagnosis and responses to medical therapy. Thyroid 7(5):755–760, 1997

Sillanaukee P: Laboratory markers of alcohol abuse. Alcohol Alcohol 31(6):613–616, 1996 9010553

Simerville JA, Maxted WC, Pahira JJ: Urinalysis: a comprehensive review. Am Fam Physician 71(6):1153–1162, 2005 15791892

Siragy HM: Hyponatremia, fluid-electrolyte disorders, and the syndrome of inappropriate antidiuretic hormone secretion: diagnosis and treatment options. Endocr Pract 12(4):446–457, 2006 16901803

Spaulding SW, Lippes H: Hyperthyroidism. Causes, clinical features, and diagnosis. Med Clin North Am 69(5):937–951, 1985 3932794

Steffes M, Cleary P, Goldstein D, et al: Hemoglobin A1c measurements over nearly two decades: sustaining comparable values throughout the Diabetes Control and Complications Trial and the Epidemiology of Diabetes Interventions and Complications study. Clin Chem 51(4):753–758, 2005 15684277

Strawn JR, Keck PE Jr, Caroff SN: Neuroleptic malignant syndrome. Am J Psychiatry 164(6):870–876, 2007 17541044

Sullivan SS, Kushida CA: Multiple sleep latency test and maintenance of wakefulness test. Chest 134(4):854–861, 2008 18842919

Surks MI, Ortiz E, Daniels GH, et al: Subclinical thyroid disease: scientific review and guidelines for diagnosis and management. JAMA 291(2):228–238, 2004 14722150

Syed Iqbal H, Balakrishnan P, Murugavel KG, Suniti S: Performance characteristics of a new rapid immunochromatographic test for the detection of antibodies to human immunodeficiency virus (HIV) types 1 and 2. J Clin Lab Anal 22(3):178–185, 2008 18484656

Theal RM, Scott K: Evaluating asymptomatic patients with abnormal liver function test results. Am Fam Physician 53(6):2111–2119, 1996 8623723

Tolmunen T, Voutilainen S, Hintikka J, et al: Dietary folate and depressive symptoms are associated in middle-aged Finnish men. J Nutr 133(10):3233–3236, 2003 14519816

Treasure J, Claudino AM, Zucker N: Eating disorders. Lancet 375(9714):583–593, 2010 19931176

Triantafyllou NI, Nikolaou C, Boufidou F, et al: Folate and vitamin B_{12} levels in levodopa-treated Parkinson's disease patients: their relationship to clinical manifestations, mood and cognition. Parkinsonism Relat Disord 14(4):321–325, 2008 18055246

U.S. Preventive Services Task Force: Screening for HIV: recommendation statement. Ann Intern Med 143(1):32–37, 2005 15998753

Vasile RG: Single photon emission computed tomography in psychiatry: current perspectives. Harv Rev Psychiatry 4(1):27–38, 1996 9384969

Vijan S: Type 2 diabetes. Ann Intern Med 152:ITC31-15, quiz ITC316, 2010

Wu AHB: Tietz Clinical Guide to Laboratory Tests, 4th Edition. St. Louis, MO, WB Saunders, 2006

Yager J, Andersen AE: Clinical practice. Anorexia nervosa. N Engl J Med 353(14):1481–1488, 2005 16207850

Young H: Guidelines for serological testing for syphilis. Sex Transm Infect 76(5):403–405, 2000 11141863

Yuan G, Al-Shali KZ, Hegele RA: Hypertriglyceridemia: its etiology, effects and treatment. CMAJ 176(8):1113–1120, 2007 17420495

Zerwekh JE: Blood biomarkers of vitamin D status. Am J Clin Nutr 87(4):1087S–1091S, 2008 18400739

Index

*Page numbers printed in **boldface** type refer to figures.*